Never 1

~ Kaler

The true story of
a young woman
who cheated death
many times
only to emerge
as a ray of light to
all who know her.

My ☆ Favorite American

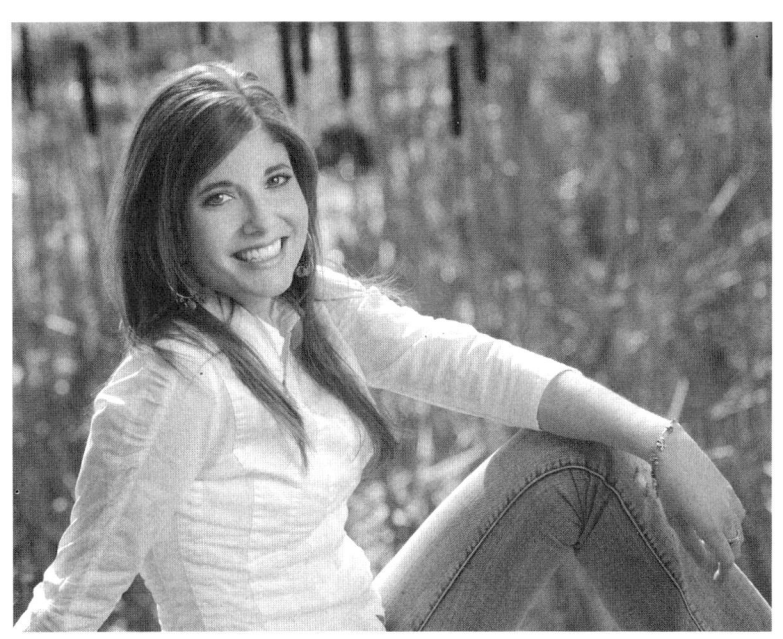

AN INSPIRING BIOGRAPHY BY
DENNIS McCLOSKEY

Dennis McCloskey

GENERAL STORE PUBLISHING HOUSE
499 O'Brien Road, Box 415
Renfrew, Ontario, Canada K7V 4A6
Telephone (613) 432-7691 or 1-800-465-6072
www.gsph.com

GSPH

ISBN 978-1-897113-87-5

Cover illustration, design and layout: Magdalene Carson / New Leaf Publication Design
Printed by Custom Printers of Renfrew Ltd., Renfrew, Ontario
Printed and bound in Canada

Library and Archives Canada Cataloguing in Publication

McCloskey, Dennis, 1948-
      My favorite American / Dennis McCloskey.
ISBN 978-1-897113-87-5
      1. Cover, Valen. 2. Polycystic kidney disease--Patients--Pennsylvania--
Biography. I. Title.
RC918.P58M34 2007   362.196'610092   C2007-907079-5

Cover Photo by Maximilian Franz, Baltimore, Maryland.

This book is dedicated to
Valen's parents,
William F. Cover III
and Pamela K. Cover;
and
Valen's kidney donor,
Sally K. Robertson

Contents

Prologue

On the afternoon of Friday, December 28, 2007, Pam Cover revealed a family secret to her twenty-four-year-old daughter, Valen. Knowing that her daughter's biography would be published in 2008, both Pam and her husband, Bill, felt the time was right to lift the veil of secrecy.

Pam learned she was pregnant with her second child. "I was totally surprised and happy, but Bill did not take the news well," she disclosed to me. "My mother had just died from PKD six months earlier, and I had the disease. Neither of us wanted to pass this terrible condition on to another child."

Pam's gynecologist suggested she get an abortion. Pam knew that abortions were illegal at the time, but her doctor assured her that this would be considered a "medical necessity" and would be approved. Pam made an appointment to terminate her pregnancy.

However, in the brief period before the scheduled date, Pam could not "come to grips" with the feeling that having an abortion was the right decision. One day, while taking a walk near her apartment, Pam spotted a woman pushing a little girl in a carriage along the sidewalk. Pam described to me the intercessional event that unfolded: "I stared at the little girl in the carriage. The woman—I assume it was her mother—never looked at me, but the little girl continued to glare at me with a penetrating look. They were across the street from me but as I passed by, the little girl and I continued to stare at each other, not breaking eye contact for one second. I knew immediately those beautiful little eyes were telling me to have this baby inside me."

The night before Pam's appointment, she read the Bible for further guidance and to "shed some light" on her situation. The next day, Bill drove her to York Hospital, where the procedure would take place. They sat in the car in the parking lot for a long time, talking. Finally, Bill said: "You don't have to have this abortion if you don't want to."

That's all Pam needed to hear. "I was so happy and relieved."

A quarter century later, they say they are thankful "for making the right decision."

The Introduction

"Although the world is full of suffering,
it is also full of the overcoming of it."
— *Helen Keller*

I don't do pain very well.

I'm not a stranger to pain, because I once had a hangnail that caused considerable distress for a few days. Three days, tops. And once, in the middle of the night, I got up to "water the lilies" and stubbed my toe on a dresser that someone had thoughtlessly placed in my path. Big toe. Right foot. Hurt for days.

I know you're feeling my pain, but that's not the worst physical hurt I have endured. A few weeks after the bruise disappeared from my lower right extremity, misfortune fell yet again. I know what you're thinking: "Hasn't this poor guy suffered enough?" Apparently not! I was lifting a heavy object (no, it wasn't on a fork!) and I heard a "snapping" sound from the general area of one of my fingers. The pinky. Right hand. Hurt like hell! I drove myself to the emergency room of our local hospital, had it x-rayed, and was told it was just a bruise. Easy for them to say. And Kilimanjaro is just a hill in Tanzania!

Valen Cover knows pain.

My twenty-five-year-old friend from York, Pennsylvania, has endured the kind of physical pain and suffering that St. Augustine called "the greatest evil." Her mountainous battle with endless distress began at age five when she suffered a seizure disorder. At ten she was diagnosed with polycystic kidney disease (PKD), one of the most common genetic life-threatening diseases that afflict 12.5 million people worldwide. Valen's grandmother died of PKD at age fifty-three, and her aunt passed away nine years ago from the illness. Valen's mother, Pam, and all of her mother's cousins have the disease, as does her thirty-one-year-old brother, Brandon, and his seven-year-old son, Branson.

When Valen's eighth-grade girlfriends were enjoying the fruits of becoming young adults and dressing up to impress boys, thirteen-year-old Valen was undergoing scoliosis back surgery and had Harrington rods inserted on both sides of her spine.

Her two diseased kidneys were removed less than two weeks before her nineteenth birthday. She spent seven agonizing months receiving dialysis treatment before undergoing a kidney transplant operation. At twenty-four, she was involved in a near-fatal motorcycle accident that temporarily broke her spirit but not her resolve to live.

I heard about Valen Cover (the "o" is long, as in "clover") in December 2005 in my capacity as a contract editor for Kingsway Financial Services. It is the parent company of more than a dozen North American insurance companies and is based in Mississauga, Ontario, in the Greater Toronto Area. Valen works for one of the subsidiary companies, Lincoln General Insurance, of York, Pennsylvania. Barb Lukawski, their Vice-President of Human Resources, contacted me in December 2005 to suggest that I write an article about "a remarkable young woman" who works as an administrative assistant in their Claims Department. (Valen was later promoted to Claims Associate in Special Projects, and in 2008 became Project Coordinator.)

It was a call that would have a profound effect on me. Before calling Valen, I spoke to a few of her colleagues to find out a bit more about her. The flattering remarks I heard regarding this young person almost bordered on hero worship: "When I think of her, tears come to my eyes," said one. "She is kind and caring," said another. A female colleague described her selfless attitude and total commitment to the PKD cause, and another spoke of her spirit, calling it a "vital spark." When a female co-worker remarked that "the world needs more Valens," I knew I had to contact this woman.

I e-mailed her on December 5, 2005, just before noon. I introduced myself and asked if I could arrange a phone interview with her for an article in the company's spring newsletter. She responded immediately. Although she was a little taken aback by the proposal, she wrote simply and modestly: "Sure, if you want to."

The phone interview took place on January 18, 2006, at 8:00 a.m., an hour after she starts work. We talked for an hour. I was impressed. At my request, she related her inventory of illnesses and operations. I was struck by her positive, confident, and optimistic spirit. She seemed infused with a divine spark. She talked of her blessings and hopes and dreams and faith and wishes. My piddling thoughts of bothersome hangnails and stubbed toes were banished forever from my mind.

I'm a writer who wears his heart on his sleeve, so it was difficult to contain my enthusiasm for this Wonder Woman. A hint of my feelings appeared on page thirteen in a bold thirty-six-point head-line of the March 2006 employee edition of the quarterly *Kingsway News,* which heralded Valen's "enduring and endearing spirit." I preceded my story with a quote by Helen Keller: "Optimism is the faith that leads to achievement. Nothing can be done without hope and confidence." I had spoken to Valen for all of sixty minutes, but I was convinced she possessed the virtues of faith and hope, in spades. My opening paragraph, under my byline, announced that I had met a truly unique and remarkable individual.

I wrote: "Once or twice in a lifetime you might meet a person with such an indomitable spirit, supreme strength, and unimaginable courage that you wonder how you got so lucky as to cross paths with her." I don't think that was verbal overkill.

Now I was dying to meet her. But that wouldn't happen for another year and a half. In the meantime, we struck up a telephone and on-line friendship that transcended age, gender, and culture. I became her mentor, friend, confidante, phone pal, and inveterate e-mail buddy. She shared her problems with me and often sought my advice. Soon, she adopted me as her "stepdad," and by now my wife, Kris, had gotten to know her so well through me that we embraced her as the daughter we never had. Now, over two years after we unofficially "adopted" her, we continue to heap upon her all the love and attention that is possible in our long-distance relationship, with us living in Canada and her in the U.S.

Before I got a chance to meet Valen in person, I had gathered enough information about her to write an inspirational-type article for a Catholic magazine, *Canadian Messenger.* It appeared in the October 2007 edition. Here is a small portion of that article, titled: "Where There Is Youth There Is Hope."

Before the age of twenty, Valen Cover had endured a litany of medical anomalies, including seizures, scoliosis,

PKD, pancreatitis, bleeding kidney cysts, a bilateral nephrectomy i.e. the removal of her two diseased kidneys, over seventy blood transfusions, extremely high blood pressure, and a successful kidney transplant. From her time in the womb when, as she puts it: "I almost didn't have a chance at life," and for the next two decades, many of her illnesses challenged some of the finest medical minds in America.

Today, she remains unbloodied and unbowed by the curveball that life has thrown at her, saying she does not dwell on the past but would rather focus on the brightest aspects of every part of her life. "As bad as things get, there is always hope," she said recently. "I consider myself blessed because I have survived all of these challenging obstacles to give others hope that they, too, can overcome all odds in life."

It is said that a wounded deer leaps the highest, and in Valen's case she possesses a spirit of such positive thought and action that she is the epitome of the phrase that "hope springs eternal in the human breast." British author Samuel Butler once wrote that young people have a marvelous facility of either dying or adapting themselves to circumstance. Valen could have retreated into a world of despair and self-pity over her circumstances, but she did not. She touched my heart when she said her life could easily be presented as a distressing tale of lost youth, lengthy hospital stays, major operations, vanishing hope, and disappearing dreams. But she will not allow those thoughts to clutter her mind. Instead, she chose to take the high road, realizing that she had been given a second chance at life, and has determined that she will turn the negatives of her life into positives by doing all she can to help find a cure to the incurable disease. She told me that a positive attitude and faith are two reasons she is alive today. "Instead of being bitter over the past, I decided to use my experiences to give strength to others with PKD," she said. "I feel that I exemplify the truth that something wonderful can come out of the most horrible experiences we endure in life."

Since her transplant on August 13, 2002, Valen said she has truly learned how valuable and precious every moment in life is. And with that resolve, she has been working tirelessly to bring about an awareness of the disease that afflicts so many. Her motivation is exemplary: "I believe that for every disadvantage there is a corresponding advantage," she said.

Today, her efforts on behalf of PKD are legendary in her community and her company. Despite holding down a full-time job, she has traveled on her vacation days to places like California to speak at an international PKD annual conference — even a fashion show in Texas — to get the message across about her battle with the disease and the need to help find a cure. For several years she has shared her story at a college lecture at the prestigious Johns Hopkins University in Baltimore. In March 2007 she addressed a gathering of the Congressional Kidney Caucus in Washington, DC. Her other efforts on behalf of the cause are legion, from forming a PKD chapter in her hometown, to organizing annual fundraising walkathons, to serving as the Campaign Chair for the 2005–2006 "Campaign for a Cure" which raised over a million dollars.

Recently I spoke to several of Valen's co-workers who used the words "courageous" and "a real leader" in describing her. I agree with their description. As a freelance journalist of over twenty-five years, a lifelong Roman Catholic, and a curious observer of the human condition, I understand that faith is an outward and visible sign of an inward and spiritual grace, and I see it in this extraordinary young woman.

It is often difficult to put into words the effect one human being has on another, but if I were to analyze my "fatherly" love for this young woman, it can be expressed in a word: hope. Mother Teresa spoke often of "creating hope and giving hope," and Valen, to my mind, manifests this spirit. But she is humble whenever this attribute is directed toward her. She does not accept lightly the mantle of "courageous heroine." She maintains she is unworthy of such adulation and certainly is not the fountain of all goodness. At times, Valen has endured the envy of others, and when this happens she gets angry. "There is nothing to be envious about," she snapped when I mentioned it. "Anyone just has to stand in my shoes for one day to know the pain and suffering I have experienced. Trust me, they would not be envious!" I pressed on, commenting on her bravery and positive outlook on life, but she was uncharacteristically testy with me, saying: "So, I understand that I must be somewhat strong to have endured everything I have. Well, so would anyone else!" She emphatically told me that she was forced to deal with her afflictions whether she liked it or not. Valen Cover is no quitter. She believes that a quitter never wins and a winner never quits. She softened her voice, saying she appreciates all the positive attention she receives. "It means the world to me," she whispered. "I keep it in my heart."

Hope is the parent of faith, and she said it was faith, hope, and the love and support of her mother and father and other members of her family and medical teams that brought her back from the abyss of death during some of the darkest hours of her life. Her humble protestations—of displaying courage in the face of death—reminded me of the words of St. Thomas Aquinas, who wrote: "Faith has to do with things that are not seen, and hope with things that are not at hand."

I sometimes joke that the trouble with young people today is that they're young. But Valen has a wisdom that belies her twenty-five years, and a mature, unselfish appreciation for the undying love she has received from others. When speaking of her parents, Bill and Pam Cover, Valen calls them her "strength," adding that she cannot begin to describe the infinite amount of love and respect she has for them. She also told me that she is humbled by the amount of love they have for one another. "Everything I do, I do for my parents and to make them proud," she said.

Today, a relatively healthy Valen says the good days outnumber the bad, even though she is not out of the woods, medically speaking. At the end of 2003, doctors found precancerous cells on her cervix. Earlier last year, she was hospitalized several times with a urinary tract infection. She is more susceptible to germs than most people and she gets colds easily. But her resolve remains strong.

I once told Valen that she is the type of person who doesn't aim for the clouds when she can aim for the stars, and I truly believe she is a rare and shooting star in our midst. My late father was a member of the Royal Canadian Air Force, whose motto is *Per Ardua Ad Astra* ("Through Adversity to the Stars"). Valen has known and conquered adversity all her young life and I know she will continue to be a role model for people of all ages as she continues to reach for the moon and the stars.

St. Paul told the Galatians, "The fruit of the Spirit is love, joy, peace, long-suffering, gentleness, goodness, and faith." When I think of those seven virtues, I think to myself: "Thy name is Valen Cover."

If any question remains of the faith and determination of this young woman, it can best be summed up in her e-mail address: **PKDwillnotbeatme@yahoo.com.**

Throughout her young life, Valen has endured ceaseless, sharp, and lasting pain, yet she has emerged like a springtime rose in bloom. At times she must have wondered if the cure was worth the pain. More likely, she adheres to poet John Dryden's sentiment that "sweet is pleasure after pain."

Valen's resilience in the face of her health issues is a constant source of amazement to me. So is her "*joie de vivre*"—her joy of living—and her ability to "put a smile on the face of the whole human race." U.S. songwriter Jay Lerner coined that phrase. I doubt that Valen has heard of this famed songbird who died in 1986, three years after she was born. But Valen's a quick learner (no pun intended) and she knows that if she smiles, others will smile back.

Her good cheer is infectious. In July 2007, I was feeling blue over the imminent death of a mutual friend. Her e-mail on that afternoon was titled: "Don't be sad, dad." She wrote sweetly and innocently: "Unfortunately, we do not always have good days and our friend is not having a good day." But in her eternal optimistic spirit, she added that he should get better as soon as he received two blood transfusions scheduled for later that day. "I spent nearly a year of 'not good days' in the hospital and stressing about it did not help. But plugging away did help!"

It was the student teaching the teacher.

She continued: "I have come to the conclusion that if we let things sadden us and continually ask 'why' and try to make sense of everything, we are wasting the precious time we have here on earth. We just need to hang in there and find strength in support of each other."

She ended her e-mail: "Cheer up! We have many rewarding days to come." This came from a woman who was given up for dead by some members of the medical community in 2002. Where, I ask myself, does such optimism come from? Deep, deep inside, no doubt. From the same inner core that's found in people like Helen Keller, who said: "Be of good cheer and do not think of today's troubles, but of the success that may come tomorrow."

It wasn't Helen Keller I was thinking about on the bright morning of Tuesday, May 8, 2007, as I peered out the tiny window of the Beechcraft 1900 airliner that would soon deliver me to Pennsylvania's Harrisburg International Airport in south-central Pennsylvania. I was hoping to spot the Three Mile Island Nuclear Generating Station near Harrisburg, but it's south of the city and we were flying in from the north, from Toronto. I had long wanted to see the plant that was best known for being the site of the worst civilian nuclear accident in U.S. history when TMI-2 suffered a partial meltdown in 1979. It would wait for another trip. And it did. I saw it up close, in a vehicle with five others, several months later. As the nineteen-seater regional aircraft flew over the Blue Ridge chain of the Appalachian Mountains and made its way toward the rich, fertile agricultural fields that surround Harrisburg, my thoughts turned to the music I was listening to on my iPod. Bruce Springsteen was singing a song of hope.

These are better days baby
These are better days it's true
These are better days
Better days are shining through

I was on my way to York, Pennsylvania, a city of 41,000 that's known as the White Rose City, twenty-three miles south-east of Harrisburg. I was on a two-day corporate newsletter assignment to interview Ed Loch, a Special Investigation Unit (SIU) employee for Lincoln General Insurance Company of York. A retired, twenty-six-year veteran of the U.S. Marine Corps, Ed had been diagnosed with Stage 4 pancreatic cancer in April 2006. He was on disability leave from Lincoln General Insurance, but was well enough to meet with me to tell his story and to deliver a message to his fellow employees to take care of their health through regular checkups. I was looking forward to meeting the former Marine who was an iconoclastic figure in the SIU field. But it was also an opportunity for me to meet, for the first time, the young woman who had touched my heart fourteen months previously. Valen and Ed were good friends and co-workers. Before I left Toronto, I had made plans to meet them both for dinner at the end of my day of interviewing and photographing Ed.

My thoughts of Ed and his disease were interrupted by "The Boss," who was now belting out "Born in the USA," his 1984 hit.

> *Born down in a dead man's town,*
> *The first kick I took was when I hit the ground ...*
> *Born in the U.S.A.*
> *I was born in the U.S.A.*

I was born in Prince Edward Island, on Canada's east coast. Not in the U.S.A. But I thought of some people I know who were. Like the Henquinets and the Clarks of Chicago; my cousins in Seattle and California; Dianne Cahill and her two boys in South Carolina; and David Egan and family, in Boston, to name just a few. And Valen — the five-foot-three, life-affirming woman whom I had grown to admire and respect for her tenacity, humor, and invincible spirit. By now I knew enough about her life-and-death struggles that I could repeat them by memory. But in all the conversations we had and all the e-mails we shared, not once did she seek sympathy. She is not a "poor me, why me" whiner. "In all my years on this planet," she once wrote, "my eyes have seen enough pain to know there are many who have it far worse than I." Her cup runneth over with the milk of human kindness. She loves a good quote and she repeats one of her favorites every chance she gets: "When God gave me lemons, I made lemonade."

> *Born in the U.S.A.*
> *I'm a cool rocking daddy in the U.S.A.*

The New Jersey singer and his E-Street Band have long been my rock favorites, and as I listened while the regional jet streaked over Valen's state of Pennsylvania, I was thinking of some of the qualities that I admired in this person who is more than three decades my junior.

Fortitude is one of her beatitudes.

This is a woman who never gives up in the face of adversity, even as a five-year-old when her tiny body was thrashing about in rhythmic convulsions on her parents' kitchen floor, the result of her first grand mal seizure. The child got up, dusted herself off, and moved on. And Valen never quit when doctors removed her two bloody, cyst-covered kidneys that were the size of footballs.

The small aircraft dipped toward the east as it made its approach to the city of Harrisburg in the Susquehanna Valley. I had yet to meet her in person, but I knew some of her best characteristics: Humility. Kindness beyond measure. Charity. Temperance. Understanding. Diligence. And an abundance of faith, hope, and love.

An unusual thought crossed my mind: Of the 300 million Americans alive today, I personally know a very small number—maybe a hundred, thanks to my writing career—but Valen surely ranks up there as one of my favorites. Hmmm. My favorite American. What a great title for a book. I thought to myself: "If I ever write her life story, that will be the title."

The plane landed and parked on the tarmac a short distance from the terminal gate. I descended the stairs ahead of a dozen other passengers and walked to the small terminal, which was sparsely populated on this Tuesday morning at 11:10. By prior arrangement, Valen had offered to meet me at the airport and drive me to the Lincoln office to meet Ed. I was a little nervous. I felt like a father meeting his grown-up adopted daughter for the first time. And in a way I was.

She spotted me at the same time I recognized her. She sprang from the airport lounge chair and bounded toward me. Her blonde-streaked hair fell to just above her waistline. She wore dark brown slacks that flared at the bottom, nearly touching the floor. Her top was a blaze of color: large, pink flowers dominated the fabric of brown, tan, white, and light green. Her fashionable attire was accented by a short necklace and gold, dangling earrings. Her smile was as broad as the mile-wide Susquehanna River that dominates the landscape in this part of Pennsylvania. I gave her a gift of a bright purple and pink boa that my wife had made especially for her. The scarf and top was a perfect match. She posed while I snapped a picture. We made our way to the parking lot, both of us chattering like old friends. Which we were. Sort of.

She eased her tiny frame behind the wheel of the company car that her boss, John Macharsky, allowed her to use to meet me. As I settled into the passenger seat, the radio came on full blast as she turned on the car engine. We both looked at each other and burst out laughing. Hall and Oates were singing "Maneater," their 1982 song about an '80s carnivorous chick.

> *Oh here she comes*
> *Watch out boy she'll chew you up*
> *Oh here she comes*
> *She's a maneater*

I pretended to reach for the door handle to make a quick exit. "Oh no, what have I got myself into?" I asked, feigning fear between fits of laughter.

> *Nothing is new, I've seen her here before*
> *Watching and waiting*
> *She's seated with you but her eyes are on the door*

We regained our composure, and soon we were on the road to her city of York. Since it was just after noon, we decided to stop for lunch before my afternoon meeting with Ed. She pulled into a favorite restaurant. Charlie Brown's Steakhouse is where she and Ed met for lunch just about every Friday. He would describe his latest medical complication, and she would listen with a sympathetic ear and offer advice or encouragement, whichever she felt he needed at that particular time. Ed could not join us. He'd had a regular round of chemotherapy the previous night and had phoned that morning to say he was not feeling well, but was looking forward to the afternoon talk with me. Valen and I babbled incessantly while we munched on a fresh salad. Our beverage of choice was lemonade, naturally.

During lunch I shared with her the thought I had while airborne and listening to the Springsteen song. She laughed at the notion of a book being written about her one day and was humbled by my suggested title.

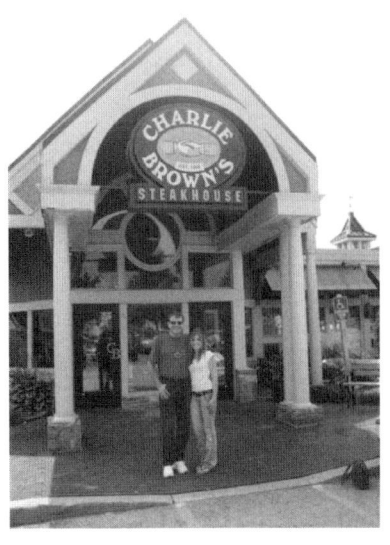

The biographer and his subject in front of their favorite York restaurant.

At 1:15 p.m. we climbed back into the company car. After fastening our seatbelts, Valen slipped the key into the ignition and the engine roared to life. Once again the radio blared and just as we did a few hours before, we turned to each other and laughed. But this time we were truly stunned. It was the sound of Springsteen. "Born in the U.S.A." My mouth was wide open. Valen's eyes were like saucers. "I don't believe it!" she exclaimed. "This is not even my car. I never listen to this station and I hardly ever hear this song!"

I suggested that a rare coincidence had just occurred. But Valen believed otherwise. "I don't believe in coincidence," she said. "Everything happens for a reason."

Maybe it does. Maybe a Canadian writer and a PKD victim from Pennsylvania were destined to meet. So that I could tell the life story of my favorite American.

2

The Early Years

*The events of childhood do not pass
but repeat themselves like seasons of the year.*
— *Eleanor Farjeon*

Every moment of every day someone dies, and every moment of every day someone is born.

On February 4, 1983, Pam Cover, nine months pregnant and a little nervous, phoned her doctor. When she explained her symptoms, including the time between contractions, it was confirmed she was in labor. She began to rush around the house in preparation for the ride to the hospital. Her husband, Bill, was getting out of the shower, and Grandma Emily, whom they call "Sis," was soon called to come over and look after six-year-old Brandon, who was in the TV room watching *Jaws II*.

"Well, Brandon, this is it. I'm going to have the baby."

Pam's only child looked away from the monstrous shark that was terrorizing the water-bound citizens of Amity. "Why? Did your water break?"

"No, I have a bloody show," Pam explained. During her pregnancy, Pam had taken her young son to Big Brother and Big Sister classes at the hospital, so she knew he would be familiar with the term that refers to the thick plug of mucus that blocks the cervical opening to prevent bacteria from entering the uterus.

"YUCK!" he exclaimed and turned his attention back to Police Chief Brody, who was warning the townspeople of the aquatic danger just when they thought it was safe to go back in the water.

Valen Elizabeth Cover came into the world at 3:22 a.m. on February 5, 1983. It was a Saturday. I remember it well. No, I wasn't there for the blessed event. (Valen good-naturedly chastised me two dozen years later for missing "the big show.") The day is fresh in my memory because I attended the funeral of my uncle Vernon

MacGuigan, in Mississauga, Ontario. Following the morning burial, family and friends gathered at the home of Vernon's brother, prominent Toronto lawyer Leo MacGuigan. One dies and one is born. The circle of life.

Members of the Cover family gathered in a hospital room in York to rejoice in the birth of Bill's and Pam's second child. When Brandon was ushered into his mother's room, she greeted him with a warm, maternal hug.

"Well, Brandon, it's a girl."

"That's exactly what I wanted," he beamed.

The Bible teaches us there is a time for everything and a season for everything under heaven. Ecclesiastes says: "There is a time to be born and a time to die . . . a time to weep and a time to laugh . . . a time to mourn and a time to dance."

As the Cover family took turns holding the eighteen-and-a-half-inch bundle of joy, there was every indication the six-pound, five-and-one-half-ounce dark-haired infant would lead a happy, normal, carefree childhood.

And she did. For five years.

The infant's father—William ("Bill") F. Cover III—takes full credit for naming the baby "Valen Elizabeth." The middle name is in honor of his mother, Emily Elizabeth, and the first name pays homage to the day that doctors *expected* the baby to be "cast naked upon the naked earth"—February 14th, St. Valentine's Day. Bill claims a variation of the name also came from a television show he and Pam were watching that year, called *Dynasty,* starring John Forsythe as Blake Carrington, the owner of an oil empire in Denver, Colorado, and Alexis, played by Joan Collins as his glamorous but cruel ex-wife who owned a rival oil conglomerate. A central character in the prime-time soap opera was their beautiful and feisty daughter, Fallon, played by Pamela Sue Martin. So, "Fallon" became "Valen," even though their newborn daughter arrived nine days before the February day that lovers traditionally express their love for each other.

The newest addition to the Cover household was a happy and contented child who waited eighteen months before taking her first steps. She loved being bathed by her mother in the kitchen sink and it was obvious her older brother doted on her.

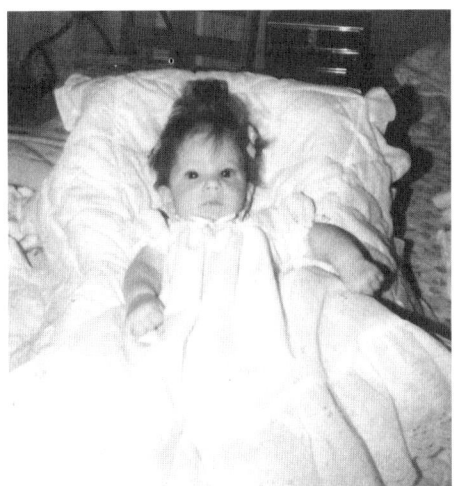

Three-month-old angel.

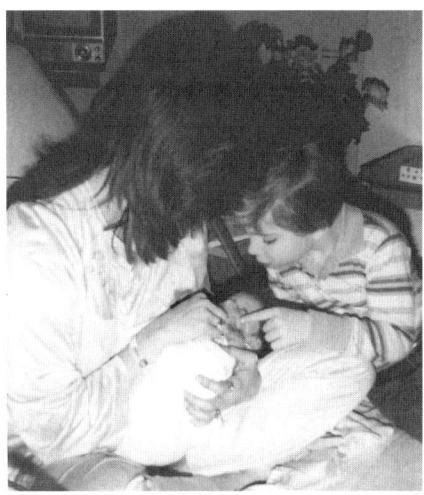

Brandon gets first peek at his new baby sister in the hospital.

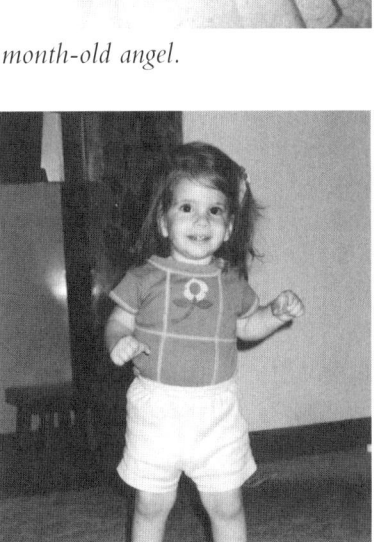

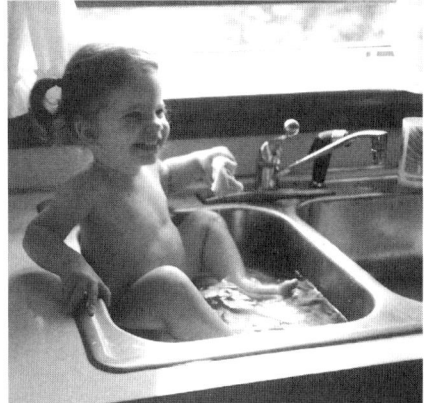

Bath time for the eighteen-month-old.

First baby steps at eighteen months.

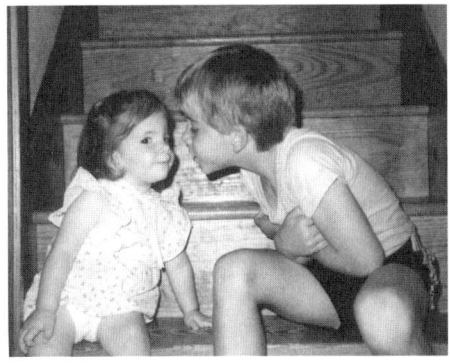

A kiss from big brother at eighteen months.

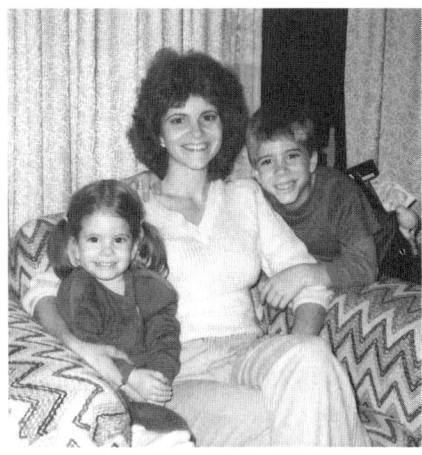

Mom (Sally Field look-alike!), son Brandon, and two-year-old daughter.

Shortly after her birth, Brandon wrote a list of thirty-four things he needed his parents for. "I need my parents for food" was his wise and practical ranking at the very top of the list, which was neatly numbered and written in pencil. Coming in at #16 was: "I need my parents for my sister." The six-year-old's gratitude at having a sister came right before "I need my parents for my dog" (#17), but after #15, "I need my parents for my toothbrush."

Notwithstanding Valen's placement nearly halfway down her brother's inventory of life requirements, and despite their age difference, the two siblings enjoyed a happy childhood together. Every owl believes its offspring is wisest, and Pam believed she had the two smartest kids on the block. This proud-as-a-peacock mom began to record her children's "silly sayings" in a journal that she started on the second day of February, 1986, when Brandon was eight days shy of his ninth birthday. According to Pam's first-born, it was Groundhog Day, "the day the goofer sees his shadow." On February 19th, three-year-old Valen was spinning around and around, and when she stopped she informed her mom she was "buzzy." On a November evening of that year, according to the diary, Valen asked her mother to sing her a "lima bean." Only Pam knew she meant "a lullaby."

Pam refers to the hardcover book of collected childish witticisms as her "Book of Silly Sayings," but not all are whimsical. Some are revealing and poignant. She printed every passage neatly and in pencil. Here is her entry for July 3, 1986:

"Valen is 3 years old. We were getting ready for bed. I tucked her in. We closed our eyes. I love to watch her with her eyes closed, her hands folded, and reciting her prayer. I said: 'Now I lay me down to sleep' and she would repeat it. I continued: 'I pray the Lord my soul to keep. Guard me Jesus through the night. And wake me with the morning light. God bless everyone. Amen. Love and kisses. Amen.' For some reason, tonight after I said 'God bless everyone' I leaned down and whispered in her ear: 'Especially Valen.' She kept her eyes closed, smiled and said: 'Especially Mommy. Amen.'"

Pam ended that particular passage with a "happy face" drawing.

The book is a treasure chest of comical, out-of-the-mouths-of-babes remarks and some unintentional "wixed-up mords." In October 1987, Pam was driving her four-year-old daughter to nursery school. It was a chilly autumn morning and Pam stifled laughter when Valen asked her to "turn on the warm air conditioning." In

January 1990, Bill was putting something together when seven-year-old Valen announced that her dad had the "indeructions" (a cross between "instructions" and "directions"). During supper in May 1990, Valen was talking about a girl at her school who got her hair cut just like Valen's. "But it's curled . . . you know, automatic." (She meant "permed.") More entries:

> **January 26, 1990:** Six-year-old Valen has started a new thing, so Brandon tells me. She sticks her tongue out. I told her if I ever saw her stick her tongue out I would smack her. A week went by. It was 9:00 p.m. Bedtime. Brandon was in a teasing mood. He made fun of her "fake" cough. Then he came running to me. "Mom, Valen just stuck out her tongue at me." In her defense, Valen argued vehemently: "I didn't try!" I replied: "Oh, right, Valen. I guess it was a spasm."
>
> **May 1, 1990:** Valen rushed in the back door from school to breathlessly relate some important news. "Jami and I went to get a drink and guess what was in the sink? You know, one of those hundred leggers!"
>
> **October 26, 1993:** Valen is guessing out loud what she will get on her first report card next week. "I think I'll get all A's and one Not-A."
>
> **November, 1995:** Coming out of a smoke-filled bowling alley with Bill and me, Valen said her coat "sniffs" (instead of "stinks").

There's more. Lots more in Pam's "Book of Silly Sayings."

The children loved special days, such as Halloween, when Pam would make costumes, and they adored Christmas and Santa Claus. The brother and his kid sister took turns writing to Saint Nick each year. What must be one of the most honest letters the jolly old fat man in the red suit has ever received came from Valen's brother at Christmas 1988. With a red felt pen, he wrote in large block letters, on behalf of himself and his five-year-old sister: "I know Valen and I have been pretty bad this year but still try to give us a couple of presents? Valen really wants a doll that walks. I'm not really sure what I want, but I know if you pick it, it will be good! Thanks. Brandon and Valen. We love you."

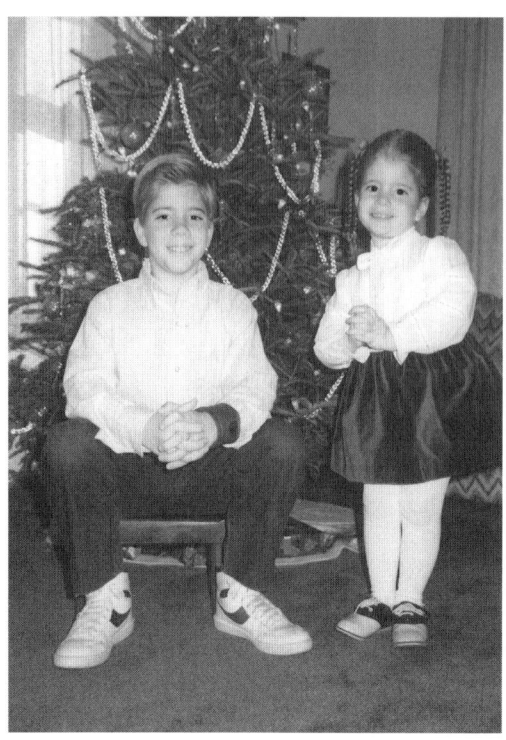

A favorite time of year for a three-year-old and her nine-year-old brother.

A few years later, it was Valen's turn to write the Santa letter. This one must rank as one of the most ingratiating letters ever sent by a child to the North Pole: "Dear Santa Claus: I would like to be surprised. The most thing that I would like is a picture of you and your reindeer. I would really like that. I would hang it on my chalkboard. If you have time please write something on my chalkboard so I will know you were here. I will always love you Santa. I will never stop. Love you forever, Valen Elizabeth Cover. P.S. Please write me back. I love you!"

Dogs were the favored pet in the household, although Valen had a guinea pig, Cinnamon, that gave birth to three healthy piglets on January 12, 1990, at 11:00 p.m. It meant a lot to Valen that she and her brother were awakened from their sleep to witness the miracle of birth. After Cinnamon delivered the third pig and cleaned the hairy offspring and then herself, its young female owner named them: Patches. Stripe. Cocoa.

Over the years, the dogs have included a West Highland Terrier (Abby); a Doberman (Molly); Dalmatian (Shelby); Sheltie (Zorro); another "Westie" (Spud); and their current dog, Zsa Zsa, a lean and excitable Hungarian Vizla. When Valen wasn't dressing her dog in cute little outfits, the preschooler liked to line up her stuffed animals on the bed and teach them. At that tender age, she had a wish to become a teacher. She had chalk, a chalkboard, and erasers in her room and would spend hours reading to them from her many books and teaching them God knows what! When she tired of playing school, she would become a cashier and count out money and change for her bedridden "customers."

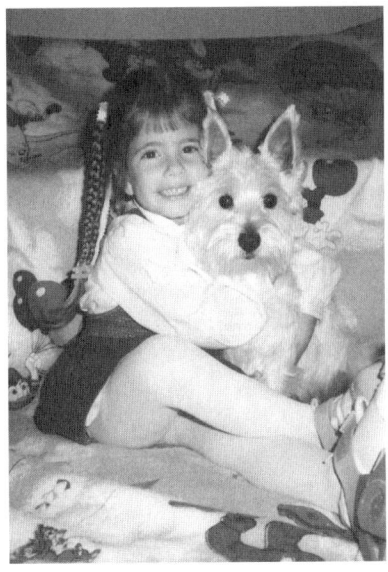

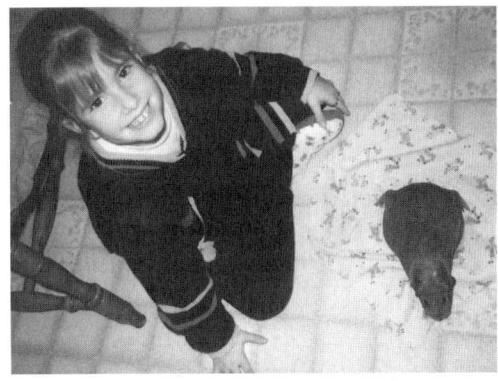

Pet guinea pig Cinnamon gives birth to triplets three weeks before Valen's seventh birthday.

Abby and her five-year-old owner.

Child psychologists like to say that children have more need of models than of critics. By the time she had reached her third birthday, Valen had three shining examples of exemplary adults to follow: Bill. Pam. And Walter.

Walter Smith and his wife, Sarah, were a retired couple who lived next door to the Cover family on York's Woodland View Drive. The families were neighbors for a dozen years, from the early '80s to the mid-'90s. The homes were practically identical; both small, brown brick, two-storey structures. The only difference was a porch on the side of Walter's house that faced the Cover home. And that's where Valen spent much of her youth. On the porch. With Walter. It was a friendship made in heaven. He loved children and he loved to teach. His young and enthusiastic neighbor loved older people and she was a willing and eager student whose curiosity knew no bounds. Long before she enrolled in kindergarten, the toddler would scurry to Walter and Sarah's and spend the day, always with her mother's knowledge, but not always with her blessing, especially when her little girl would return home for supper with her stomach full of pie made from raspberries and strawberries picked in the Smiths' backyard. "I was a little porker back then," Valen would recall two decades later. "I would eat at Walter's and then come home and eat."

When she wasn't eating bowls of sliced apples offered by Sarah, Valen would be taught reading and arithmetic by Walter. He was over sixty-five when Valen was born and was retired from his factory job where he had worked on an assembly line. "He was a very smart man," Valen recalled. "When I started school, I already knew

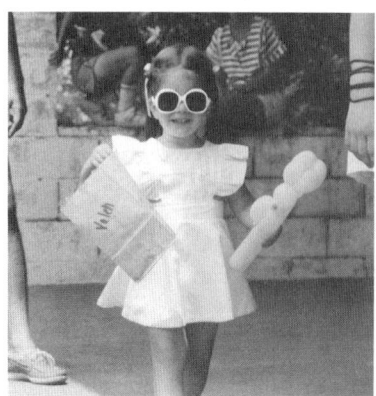

She loved sunglasses—even at age three.

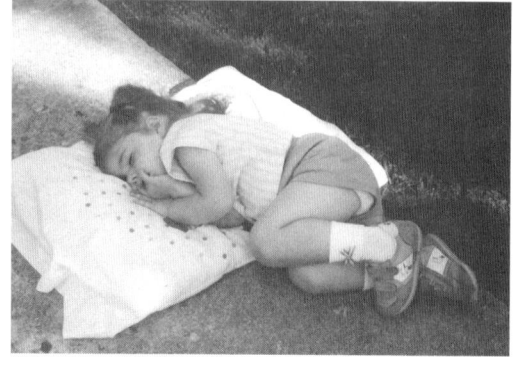

Napping on the sidewalk at age three in front of the family home.

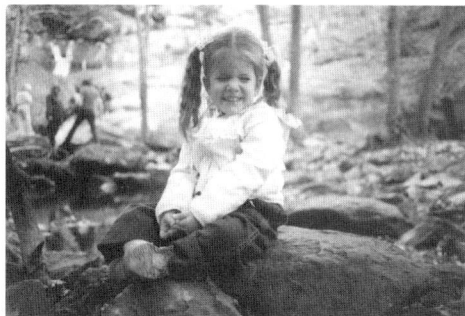

Three-year-old Valen playing on the rocks at Cunningham Falls State Park, Maryland.

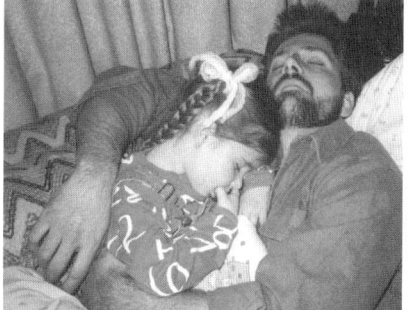

Napping inside the family home at age five, with dad.

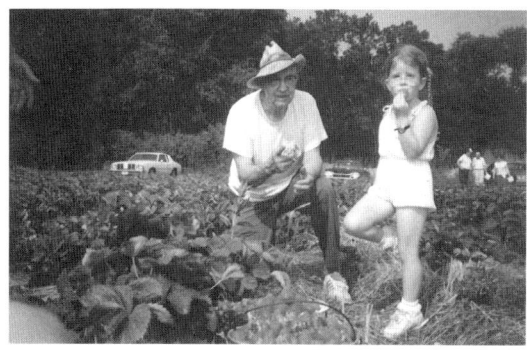

Walter picking strawberries with his five-year-old neighbor.

how to add, subtract, multiply, divide, do long division, and short division. Walter taught me everything they taught in first grade. It was pretty cool."

The tree-lined neighborhood was quiet and safe. As a tot, Valen would scamper to the sidewalk in front of her house, dragging a pillow behind her. There, with Pam looking out the window at her young charge, Valen would curl up on the cement and take a nap, sucking not on her thumb but on two fingers—the middle and ring finger.

Valen and her parents are quick to emphasize that Walter never wanted to be alone with Valen. "And he wasn't, ever!" Bill assured me. "Walter was very careful about that. He — and we — didn't want anything weird thought about him. We were very lucky to have someone like him." Pam described their neighbor as a patient and kind man. "Valen and Walter just bonded really well. Valen was enthusiastic about learning and she kept coming back and he liked that."

To this day, Valen cannot fully explain the special connection they enjoyed. "He was like a grandfather. He had a huge impact on my life." She believes it is why she bonds so well with older people today. Valen conceded that her peers find this hard to comprehend. "I spent my childhood learning from an older person and that is why I like to learn from my elders today."

She admitted she was a "different" child in that she did not want to play with other children her age. She stayed by her mother's side, and if her parents had friends over for dinner or for an evening, Valen preferred to sit with the adults and not their children. "I didn't want to play with the kids; I wanted to hang out with the adults and stay up late." She acknowledged it's probably uncommon, but she justifies it by saying it's how she grew up. "You adapt to your surroundings, and I was with adults a lot when I was young. An older man taught me things that came in handy later on in life."

Walter and Sarah moved from the neighborhood when Valen was a pre-teen and she was saddened by Walter's death on Sunday, April 27, 2003. He was ninety.

I contacted Walter's grandson, Mark McGuire — who knew the Covers when Valen was an infant — to get another take on the relationship between Valen and his grandfather. Mark, who is thirty-three, lives in Massachusetts, and is profoundly deaf, wrote in an e-mail that Valen has a special place in his heart that was nurtured by his grandfather. "The kindness that my grandfather showed other people has rubbed off on Valen," he explained. "This sweet, charming young lady can be annoying at times, and can hound you like there is no tomorrow, but there is a kindness in her that comes, in part, from her parents and partly from my grandfather."

Mark has lived in eight states in fourteen years. He wrote to me from his current home in Cape Cod, where he resides with his parents. He got to know Valen through occasional visits to his grandparents' house on Woodland View Drive, where he would join the youngster and oldster in a game of Old Maid or the board game Uncle Wiggly. The visits were few and far between and became even more so when Mark moved from York to attend Arizona State College, and his grandparents moved to a retirement village a few miles from their home. But he does not hide his feelings for the person he calls "the girl next door in my life." He admitted he loved her then and loves her now and acknowledged it was with sadness that he saw less and less of her as he moved farther away, including a stint in Alaska. He acknowledged they keep in touch, thanks to the efforts of Valen, but very long stretches of time will pass without seeing her.

"When I returned from Alaska, we went for a walk. Just the two of us. We talked; we were a little nervous because of all the time that had passed. But we knew there was still a bond that never went away." He mentioned with fondness the times Valen would track him down and, with the help of his mother, arrange for them to meet and spend a few hours together, walking and talking. He wrote of being with Valen some time ago as she drove and used hand signals to communicate with him while talking on her cell phone, all the while giggling and laughing with the same carefree spirit he saw in her a long time ago as a very young child.

Mark was neither giggling nor laughing when he heard from Valen in the fall of 2006. There had been an extra-long period of time between correspondences. They had a lot of catching up to do. Valen told him of her kidney transplant in 2002. "My world shattered," Mark wrote in his e-mail. "I did not have a clue she had PKD. I was devastated that no one had told me. When I learned that she nearly died in the hospital one night, I knew I was fortunate to be talking to her again." He was aware that she was not a healthy girl, but no one, not even Valen, burdened him with news of her illnesses. He arranged to meet her after that call in 2006 and when he did, he discovered that she was still the same "smiling, annoying, happy, beauty I had always known."

Valen's PKD wasn't the only illness Mark was not aware of.

Her first seizure came almost without warning on Thursday, September 1, 1988, at age five.

Four days earlier, Brandon had felt his little sister's hand and mentioned to his mother that it felt very warm. Pam took her daughter's temperature and was shocked to see it was 102°. She gave her a Children's Tylenol. At bedtime, her temperature was lower, but she gave her another Tylenol. The next day was Orientation Day at the school Valen would be attending. She was starting kindergarten. Her temperature was a normal 98.6°. She complained about her head hurting. Her mother thought it was "butterflies" in her stomach. Valen was very happy and excited about the prospect of starting school. She ate breakfast and lunch but very little supper, just picking at a summer sausage sandwich.

Wednesday, August 31st, was an exciting day in the Cover household. Valen went to kindergarten class for the first time, from 12:30 p.m. to 3:30 p.m. She loved it. She was ready for a lifetime of learning. However, her lack of appetite was a growing concern to her parents. On the first day of school, she ate very little cereal for breakfast, a few bites of half of a peanut butter and jelly sandwich for lunch, and some popcorn. She ate no supper but felt well enough to be taken for a visit to see her aunt and cousins, whom she had not seen in over a year.

Valen woke up at her usual time of 7:30 a.m. on Thursday, September 1st. She bounded into the kitchen and wished everyone a good morning. She was one happy little girl. She approached her mother and leaned on her shoulder as Pam ate her morning cereal. They talked about what they would do that morning before school started at 12:30. Moments later, Valen said calmly and softly: "Mommy, my head hurts."

"Probably because you are hungry," suggested Pam. "I'll cook you an egg for breakfast."

Valen repeated her mild complaint.

Pam glanced up at her little girl just as Valen placed her tiny hand on her forehead and cried out once more that her head hurt. This time it was a shrill scream. Pam leaped from her chair just as Valen fell to the floor. Stunned and perplexed, she looked at her daughter for a split second before realizing something was terribly wrong. Valen's eyes were now closed. Her muscles became rigid for about twenty seconds, and then her body flopped back and forth with uncontrolled muscle contortions. Her face and lips became white and her eyes rolled toward the top of her head.

Pam was terrified. She had no idea what was happening to her child.

Both of Valen's arms shot up violently over her head and her back arched furiously. It was a horrible sight. She was like a child possessed.

Valen was having a grand mal seizure, the worst of three known types of seizure. It was her first grand mal. It would not be her last. They would continue at sporadic intervals — sometimes on the toilet, sometimes at school in the middle of a class — until she was thirteen years old.

On the morning of her premiere seizure, Valen lost consciousness momentarily. After a minute or so, the incident ended. She lay on the floor, moaning. Pam sat her up on the floor and cradled her in her arms for several minutes. Valen was in a daze. For a few more agonizing minutes, she appeared drowsy and confused. She had taken on a dusky appearance, the result of a decreased blood oxygen level due to her impaired breathing during the seizure.

When everything was calm, Pam called her doctor. He was not in, but she talked to his partner, who confirmed that Valen had suffered a seizure and should be taken to the hospital's emergency room. Bill was at work. Pam knew she was in no condition to drive. She called her mother-in-law, Emily, and asked her to come pick them up right way.

Pam placed the telephone receiver on the cradle. Valen's lips had now turned a bluish-purple color. Her face was now chalk white. But she was very, very calm. "What's wrong, mommy?"

At the hospital, she was immediately examined in the Emergency Room and given a CAT scan. At noon she ate a hamburger and fries. At 1:00 p.m. she was given an electrocardiogram (ECG). Later that afternoon the little patient was discharged from the hospital.

That evening, Valen ate Lipton noodle soup. Bill, Pam and Brandon had leftover chicken corn soup. Life was slowly returning to normal at the little brown, brick house on Woodland View Drive. But their world would never be the same.

British author William Golding wrote that childhood is a disease; a sickness that you grow out of. Valen Cover should be so lucky. She eventually grew out of childhood, but she brought along with her a litany of illnesses and disease that would haunt her throughout her high school years and into adulthood. At age five, the seizures were the first of a series of ailments. But the first was not the worst. More grievous and life-threatening bodily disorders would handicap the little girl who loved dogs and Santa Claus and who wanted to be a kindergarten teacher.

While not life-threatening, the seizures were a hindrance and a big concern, not knowing when one could occur. Valen has no recollection of what transpired during the seizures but she remembers vividly the pain in her head prior to the first grand mal until she fell to the floor in an unconscious heap. On another occasion, she was sitting with her mother on the large, lavender toy box in Valen's bedroom, reading a book. She dropped the book, had a petit mal seizure, picked up the book in less than thirty seconds and continued to read. Her mother told her about it a week later.

Other episodes were much more serious. Like the one on Sunday, July 25, 1993, when ten-year-old Valen joined her father for a bicycle ride.

She slept in until nearly nine a.m., and the first thing she did, as part of her morning routine, was to take her seizure medicine, which included Tegretol. Skipping breakfast, she and her dad hopped on their bikes just before 9:30 and rode for awhile before taking a ten-minute rest. Later, they stopped for a visit at a friend's house and stayed nearly forty-five minutes before leaving for the four-mile trip home. There were some hills along the way, and the temperature was 86°F with high humidity. As soon as they parked the bikes and entered the house, Valen lay on the sofa and told her mother she did not feel well. Five minutes later she had a grand mal seizure. Her eyes thrust upward and she made a snorting sound through her nose. Her head tilted to one side and her body twitched several times. Her legs and arms jerked very hard, but just once. Then, her eyes opened very wide and she regained consciousness. The seizure had lasted thirty seconds.

Despite the seriousness of the seizure disorder and not knowing when the next one could occur, and where Valen and her parents would be, Bill and Pam were determined not to let the ailment interfere with their child's growth and development. They immersed her in regular childhood activities, such as preschool plays and coloring contests. She played the role of Cinderella in a *Salute to Walt Disney* production at Hayshire Nursery School.

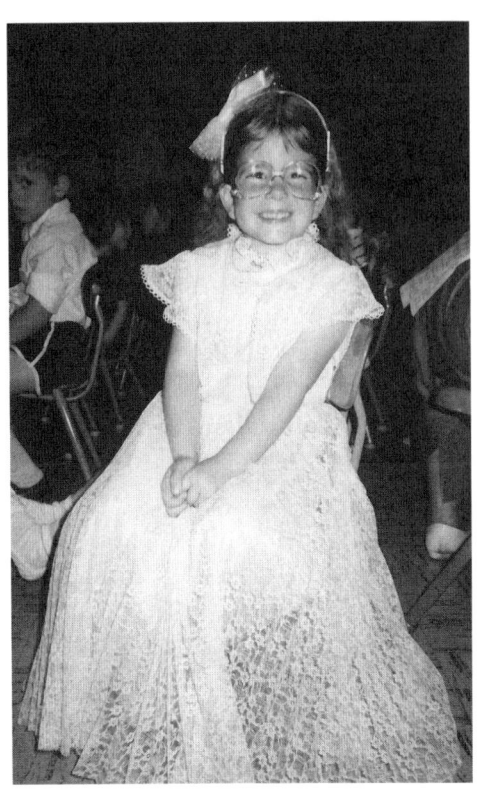

Playing the lead role of Cinderella in a production at Hayshire Nursery School.

Young Valen loved to color, taking great pride in staying inside the lines. She subsequently won oodles of community and pre-school coloring contests. Her life was as normal as possible under the circumstances. She joined the family on winter sledding outings and bowling nights, although there were early indications that sports would not be her forte. On January 2, 1989, a nearly six-year-old Valen joined her mom, dad, and brother at a York bowling alley. In one game, the scoring sheet indicated a total tally of three for Valen and eighty-one for Brandon. Pam got 107, and Dad won the game with a respectable score of 174 that included four spares and four strikes. Valen may have lost the game, but her humor won the night. Next to her name she drew a large heart and beside her brother's name, she penciled a broken heart.

Grandma Emily Cover retired from her job in 1984, so she had plenty of time to babysit her two grandchildren. Emily described Valen as a very typical child who loved having her mother do her hair in braids and pigtails. For Christmas 1988, pictures in the family photo album reveal that Pam French-braided her daughter's hair and intertwined it with red and green ribbons.

Valen, who to this day calls her grandmother "awesome," liked having Emily join the family on cookouts and excursions to the beach. A favorite family destination was Ocean City, Maryland, a popular vacation spot on the east coast because of its white, sandy beaches and world-famous boardwalk. OC, as the locals call it, is bordered on the south by Virginia and the north by Delaware and provides the only seacoast in Maryland. Valen still has a special affinity for water in any and all forms: Rain. Lakes. Rivers. Oceans.

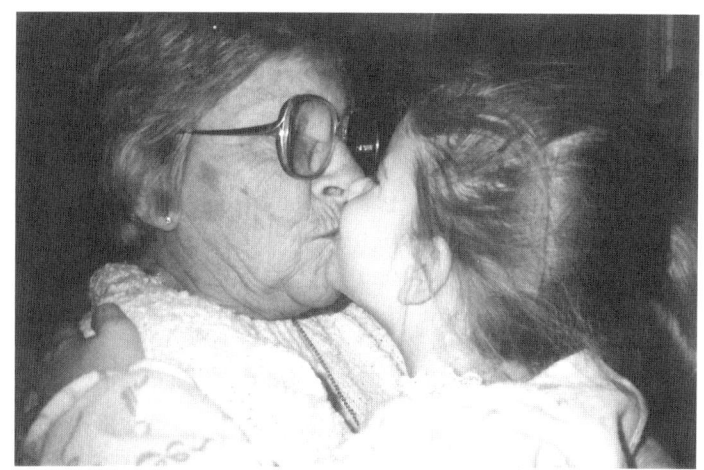

Grandma Emily gets a kiss from her two-year-old granddaughter.

Next to holidays and trips to the beach, Valen's other favorite activity was going to school, where she adored her teachers but not necessarily her classmates. "I never wanted to play with kids when I was a kid," she would admit as an adult. Her mother said she came by it honestly, meaning she, too, adored school but abhorred her fellow classmates and the scorn and ridicule they heaped upon her. Pam suffered from scoliosis and wore a Milwaukee brace for a period of time at school. The unattractive piece of equipment is a correctional back/body brace worn to treat the lateral curve of the spine in scoliosis. "Kids treated me differently," Pam told me. "They made me feel unequal. They were cruel. I didn't want to talk to anyone or look at anyone because I wasn't like them."

Perhaps still under the spell of Walter and the company of grown-ups, Valen was passed from kindergarten into first grade at the end of the 1988–89 school year at Hayshire Elementary School with mostly E's for Excellent. Her kindergarten teacher, Miss Whittaker, called her a "cooperative and enthusiastic" student. "Having Valen in my class this year has been a delight," she wrote. "She has done so well for me. I will miss her."

In first grade, under the tutelage of Mrs. D. LaVana, Valen progressed normally despite suffering a seizure during class one day. Mrs. LaVana's first-period comments referred to Valen as "a conscientious student [who] is very eager to learn."

Valen's achievement record in the second and third grades was also satisfactory, and her teachers were pleased with her progress and her eagerness to learn. While she missed only thirteen days from school in second grade, Valen—who got her first haircut at age seven—felt chubby, blaming her seizure medicine, Tegretol, for the extra pounds that plagued her throughout her early school years. "I had low self-confidence," she confided.

Her self-assurance may have been lacking, but she was number one in the personality department, according to her teachers. "Valen continues to be a delight in the classroom," wrote her second-grade teacher, Mrs. Weikel, who also commented on her excellent creativity, work habits, and shining personality. "I really enjoy my daily conversations with Valen. She is always pleasant and smiling."

The next year, in third grade, a few more B's and A's appeared on the Elementary Progress Report Card, but it was in fourth grade at North Hills Elementary School that the girl with braces on her teeth hit her stride with plenty of top marks. Her teacher, Mrs. Figdore, seemed to take a shine to her young student. Her written First Marking Period comments for the 1992–93 school year were glowing: "Valen: a great writer named Thomas Carlyle once wrote: 'Have a purpose in life, and having it, throw into your work such strength of mind and muscle as God has given you.'You have a lot of 'strength of mind,'Valen. I want you to continue to use it well."

Henry Adams wrote that teachers affect eternity; they never know where their influence stops. It could be that Mrs. Figdore provided the spark that lit a flame in Valen, both academically and creatively.Valen recalled that Mrs. Figdore took her to the park one day for lunch. "She didn't do that with other students," she said proudly.

She admits to having liked a lot of her teachers. And they loved her. Fifth grade was the year the flower bloomed, if Valen's teachers were any judge. "Valen has made tremendous strides since the beginning of the year in terms of her self-confidence," wrote Mrs. King in the First Marking Period of 1994. By Third Period, she wrote that Valen continued to set high standards for herself. "Valen should always be encouraged to focus on her strengths as she tends to be very self-critical and does not give herself enough credit, sometimes." By the Fourth Marking Period, Mrs. King's comments were over the top, declaring that her prized student was "extremely well-motivated, self-directed with very good study skills, and an exceptional student who always gives 110%." In an understatement, Mrs. King added that she truly enjoyed having Valen in her class.

When Valen was ten going on eleven, she wore oversized, silver-framed glasses that grazed her chubby cheeks. Her thick, curly, reddish-blonde hair stopped just above her shoulders. She was developing a fashion sense that would be refined and would define her in adulthood. The style-conscious girl-child liked to wear bright, voguish clothes. A favorite top was a purple blouse with ruffled collar and bow, accented with a black velvet choker around her neck with dangling silver heart and peace symbols. Bill and Pam's little girl was beginning to blossom. On a red and black cardboard poster, she penned a brief biography in multi-colored sentences, writing that she inherited her academic ability from her dad and her artistic talent from her mom. "I enjoy learning," she added in purple lettering. And in blue she wrote: "I put a lot of thought in everything I do." Red now: "I continuously strive to be the best that I can be — for myself as well as for my parents." She would repeat that last sentence to me, almost verbatim, fourteen years later.

Her last year at North Hills Elementary School appeared to be a turning point in the young girl's life. She received the Principal's Award certifying a straight-A average.

Her future was full of promise.

Things were looking up.

Then her world came crashing down.

Valen was diagnosed with autosomal dominant polycystic kidney disease (ADPKD).

The devastating news came from doctors at Pediatric Care of York, on Joppa Road. During a routine visit to the family's pediatrician, Dr. Nussbaum, Valen's blood pressure was taken. It was not usual practice at that time to take every child's blood pressure, partly because it's generally so low in children. High blood pressure is one of about ten symptoms of ADPKD, so when it was learned Valen's blood pressure was exceptionally high at 160/140, further tests were conducted because of her family's history of PKD.

In 2007, Valen and I visited the medical center where she first learned she had PKD. We met with Dr. Sean Campbell, who was not her doctor at the time of the diagnosis, but became her pediatrician shortly thereafter. A mild-mannered, fair-haired man, the father of two teenagers knew he wanted to become a doctor at the age of two. He has been at the York facility for sixteen years.

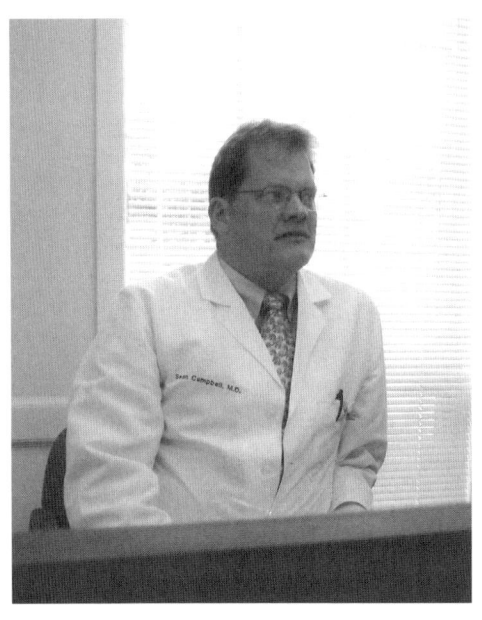

Dr. Sean Campbell, Valen's former pediatrician in York.

"I remember Valen like the back of my hand," he said fondly. "We hit it off right away." He pulled out her file and leafed through the charts for reference. He reminded us that PKD is not uncommon among young children, so when it was discovered that Valen's blood pressure was so high, further tests were taken that led to the PKD diagnosis. Now the procedure is routine. "You are the reason we now check children's blood pressure," he said, looking at the young pioneer across the desk of his small office. "Because of you, thousands of children have had their blood pressure taken here."

The affinity between doctor and patient becomes very obvious when the two talk about seeing each other around town, at the local Wal-Mart and once at a music festival in Harrisburg. Dr. Campbell spoke of the many difficulties Valen faced while she was his patient, including scoliosis back surgery. "She had the usual illnesses that every kid gets and she also went through the trials and tribulations of navigating teenage life." He called her a "great kid" who suffered a lot of "whammies," yet she was strong and always had such a big smile. "She hasn't changed at all. She still has the same beaming smile and is a real Joy Bell."

Dr. Campbell rarely thinks of himself as a lifesaver but rather one who is able to alter the life of a troubled or sick youngster. And his practice goes far beyond prescribing medicine or ordering tests. He also dispenses fatherly advice. He spoke of a young female former patient who had dropped out of school and was drifting aimlessly. He "nagged" her to go back to school, and to his delight she did and received a high school diploma. "This teen did not have a baby and she did not go to jail," he said, proudly. "That's as good as it gets for me."

His compassion became even more evident as we rose to leave his office following the evening visit. I stood in the doorway as Dr. Campbell rounded his desk and embraced his former patient with a long and tender hug. His eyes were tightly shut and I could clearly sense the genuine care, kindness and goodness in this children's doctor.

The disheartening diagnosis of PKD was a bitter pill for everyone to swallow, especially for Pam, the carrier of the disease. But it was not a complete shock. The disease was rampant in Pam's family and she knew only too well if one parent has the disease, there is a fifty percent chance the disease will pass to a child, and that both males and females are equally affected. PKD is an equal opportunity disease: it affects men, women and children — regardless of age, race or ethnic origin. According to PKD Foundation officials, it does not skip a generation.

Bill and Pam knew the statistics: PKD is one of the most common life-threatening genetic diseases, affecting more people than Down's syndrome, cystic fibrosis, muscular dystrophy, and sickle cell anemia — combined. They were only too well aware that ADPKD causes fluid-filled cysts to grow on the kidneys, and over time these cysts multiply and grow, causing kidney failure in fifty percent of cases. The numbers are equally disturbing: an estimated 600,000 Americans and 12.5 million newborns, children and adults — worldwide — fight PKD every day. The stark reality is that there is no treatment or cure for PKD. Dialysis and transplantation are the only treatment options for kidney failure.

But there was a glimmer of hope for their child. Although ADPKD affects one in 500 worldwide, it is often called the adult polycystic kidney disease. Symptoms usually develop between the ages of thirty and forty. Pam was thirty-seven years old when Valen was diagnosed. Pam had the disease, but so far her kidneys appeared healthy. There was hope their daughter could live a normal childhood, and, who knew, with medical advancements maybe there would be a cure before more fluid-filled cysts developed on both of her kidneys.

Hope springs eternal in the human breast.

Life resumed as normal as possible at 439 Woodland View Drive.

Valen thrived at school, earning a place on the Distinguished Honor Roll in the sixth and seventh grades at Central York Middle School, on North Hills Road. When the family moved to a sprawling home at 2450 Fairway Drive, Valen enrolled in West York Junior High School and continued to flourish. Her grades reflected her attitude: straight A's in English, Geography, Math, Science, Keyboarding, Art, and Home Economics. Teacher comments mirrored her stellar academic achievements: "Self-motivated. Very Creative. Conscientious student. Pleasure to have in class."

Art was her newfound creative outlet. She collected a number of awards and certificates: The Principal's Award for a lobby art display in 1994; a Language Arts Excellence Award the next year; and in that same year an award of distinction for outstanding performance and exceptional achievement; and, written in pen, presumably by a teacher: "Overall great attitude." Her art included many forms, as evidenced by a certificate for "Outstanding Achievement in Art" for a texture/pattern design contest.

Valen loved the new house on Fairway Drive. It was a three-storey home situated within the lush greens of Honey Run Golf Club. The house featured a wraparound deck and lots of windows to allow natural light to flood the large foyer. Valen was given one of two master bedrooms, and she especially loved the finished basement where she could hang out with her friends.

Youth are resilient, and most are forgiving and understanding. Even Valen was becoming accustomed to—and accepting of—her medical anomalies. Not liking them, but living with them. In 2007 she sent me one of her favorite quotes by nineteenth-century humorist Josh Billings: "Life consists not in holding good cards but in playing those you hold, well." In the mid 1990s, the preteen was just playing the cards God dealt her. And playing them well.

In his 1978 song, "The Gambler," Kenny Rogers warns: "You got to know when to hold 'em, know when to fold 'em / Know when to walk away and know when to run." It's a song about the secret to survival. Valen Cover is not one to run and hide, although she may have flirted with the notion, once. In eighth grade, the thirteen-year-old wrote a nine-stanza poem titled, "Growing Up and Moving On." It began:

> As the curtains close on my years at Junior High,
> I just sigh, smile, and say oh my.
> In these two years I've been through so much,
> That sometimes I just want to hide in a hutch.

She certainly did not win any accolades for this poem, but it was fraught with emotion. The middle stanzas informed the reader of the latest, darkest, and cruelest chapter of her young life. Incredibly, but true to form, the poem ended with a positive tone:

The curtains now will open again on my years to come at the High
School,
Which is going to be so very cool.
Even though I'm now going to be at the bottom of the totem pole,
Where I'll probably feel as small as a tadpole.
Soon I'll be on top again,
Standing at graduation where on my face there will be a big, happy grin.
I am so very excited for this day,
Where my future will be on its lovely way.

In the middle verses, not printed here, she spelled out in plain English but uneven iambic pentameter how her school year was interrupted for several months at the halfway point by debilitating back surgery. Valen had developed scoliosis, an abnormal lateral and rotational curvature and deformity of the spine.

Eighth Grade didn't start out too bad,
Towards the middle of the year I became very sad.
Scoliosis surgery, wow that's what I said!
I felt like curling up and never coming out of bed.

At thirteen, Valen was on the cusp of young adulthood. She and her female classmates twittered over the cute guys in class, but deep inside she was still battling her demons of self-confidence. While she worked on building up her inner self, she was also coping as bravely as possible with three major physical abnormalities: a seizure disorder, a life-threatening kidney disease, and scoliosis.

I know what you're thinking: "Hasn't this poor girl suffered enough?"

Apparently not.

This was just the beginning.

3

The Terrible Teen Years

"I was frightened more than words can say,
Again and again every night, I would pray."
—Valen Cover, "Growing Up and Moving On,"
1996 poem

Every life and every childhood is filled with sickness and pain. With scoliosis, some degree of the distressing disorder is found in approximately ten percent of all adolescents, but less than one percent have curves that require medical attention. Valen was among this miniscule number, and in her case the curvature was progressing. Curves less than twenty degrees are not usually treated, and for children or adolescents whose curves progress to thirty degrees, bracing may be required. Valen's curvature was well beyond that mark. It had grown into a severe S-curve and it was pressing dangerously into her lungs. Her orthopedic surgeon scheduled the surgery to correct the problem.

A curvature that appears between the ages of ten and thirteen, near the beginning of puberty, is called adolescent idiopathic scoliosis. Various causes of scoliosis have been implicated, but it is poorly understood, and there is no consensus among scientists as to the cause. Contrary to popular belief, it does not come from poor posture, sleeping on an old mattress, diet, or carrying a heavy book bag exclusively on one shoulder. In a medical breakthrough in April 2007, researchers at Texas Scottish Rite Hospital for Children identified the first gene associated with idiopathic scoliosis.

In preparation for the surgery, the Cover family was instructed to have Valen contribute her blood so she would receive her own blood during the operation. A pint was taken each time she donated her blood at the hospital, but after one particular session she became very ill when she got home. An ambulance was called, and doctors realized her blood level had dropped to an alarmingly low level. It was decided to take just a half pint next time, because a full pint was too much for her body to give up in one sitting. Pam remembers taking her home from the hospital after she recovered. "I made chipped beef for supper that evening," she remembered. "She felt better after eating the chipped beef!"

Pam also recollected that the surgery was "huge." She described seeing her daughter in the recovery room. "The incision went from the base of her neck to the lower part of her spine. It was held together with staples. There was also a large six-inch incision on the right side where they removed bone from her hip to fuse her spine."

The spinal fusion was performed to straighten the spine and then to fuse the vertebrae together to prevent further curvature. To achieve fusion, the involved vertebrae were exposed and scraped to promote growth. The bone harvested from her hip was grafted to the vertebrae so when it healed it would form one solid bone mass, and the vertebral column would become rigid to increase the likelihood of fusion. In order to maintain the proper spinal posture before fusion occurred, two stainless steel rods were implanted along the spine and attached to the vertebrae by hooks and screws. The metal rods, called Harrington rods and named after the inventor Paul Harrington, aren't needed once fusion is complete, but these will never be removed from Valen's back. The Harrington rods are now obsolete as newer and more effective types of spinal instrumentation have been developed since Valen's operation, which left a permanent scar down the entire length of her back.

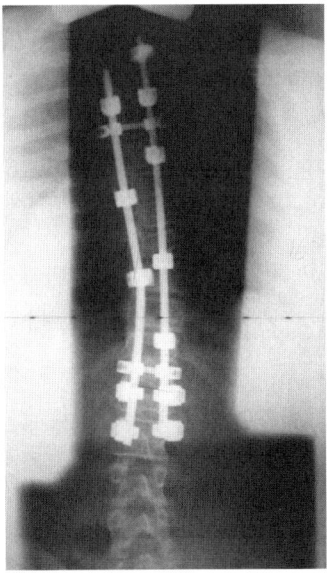

An x-ray of Valen's spine after scoliosis surgery shows permanent Harrington rods in her back.

Getting her hair washed in the hospital by Mom after scoliosis surgery.

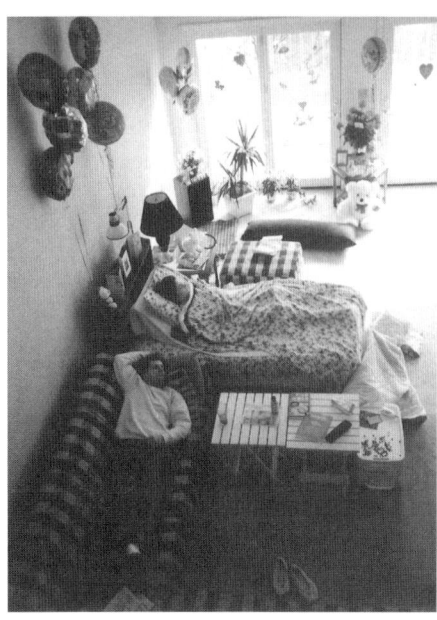

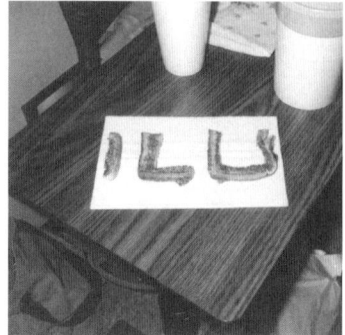

Dad carves up French toast to show his love for his sick daughter.

Father and daughter sleeping in the makeshift bedroom of the family's living room after Valen's scoliosis surgery.

To Valen, this latest hindrance in her life was another major setback. Full recovery would take six months, so arrangements were made to have her home-schooled. That wasn't necessarily the kiss of death for a young girl who loved school but not her critical schoolmates. Her middle school teachers came to the house regularly to help Valen keep up with the work and her classmates' progress. While she recovered, she immersed herself in her schoolwork, continued to achieve A's in most subjects, and managed to stay on the Distinguished Honor Roll. She credits the role of her teachers at West York Junior High for their dedication to her. *It worked out great, the teachers were really cool,* she wrote in her reflective, coming-of-age poem, "Growing Up and Moving On." *They were so wonderful to me. They filled my heart with such wonderful glee.*

The written words were harmonious from a girl who was fast becoming a realist. But discord followed when she returned to school. Sadly, she discovered that her old friends had abandoned her for other companions. Before the end of each class, she had to leave the room prior to the bell's ringing because it would be unsafe for her to be in a hallway full of active teenagers. A classmate was asked to carry her books. It was an awkward time for Valen. She was struggling with her self-esteem; she wanted to fit in, to be viewed as "normal," but she stuck out like a sore thumb. To make matters worse, the friend who carried her books deserted her, because she felt "stupid" carrying Valen's book bag around the school.

When I asked Valen a decade later to reflect on that hurtful period of time, she admitted it was very difficult. "The kids were cruel. There were so many cliques. It was all about what they were wearing. Few were nice to me."

The twenty-four-year-old paused to refresh her memory. She ignored the red recording light on the microcassette tape recorder that I had set beside her. She continued her mild rebuke. "It's all about trying to fit in, but that takes away the real purpose of going to school, which is to get a good education and learn to form sincere and lasting relationships with your peers. It shouldn't be about dwelling on the material things like who has the nicest clothes or who has a boyfriend and who doesn't. I think it's more stressful for girls."

Often a journalist's job is to be the listener, not the questioner. I remained unobtrusive. I sensed it was a cathartic moment for her. The pitch and intonation of her voice rose slightly. "I was the girl who carried a pillow because of my back surgery. I was the girl with the kidney problems who couldn't participate in gym class. 'Don't even bother to ask her to play baseball, because she can't twist her back so she can't use a bat.' It was all super annoying."

As a thirteen-year-old who didn't want to draw attention to her infirmities, Valen instinctively knew her classmates were just trying to fit in. But for her it was more difficult. She did not belong to the "in" crowd, so she was abandoned by her peers. She felt painfully alone, yet she incisively wrote that she was "sad, at first" but eventually came to see it as her call. "This call showed me that my old friends really weren't true friends and I'm happy that I moved on . . ."

And move on she did.

She dived headlong into her studies, and two months before the end of the 1997 school year, her final report card was filled with flattering comments from her teachers. She achieved A's in just about every course of study. And she was becoming a budding poet. One of her poems appeared in a 441-page, hard-cover book of poems titled *A Celebration of Pennsylvania's Young Poets, 1997*. It is titled "Parents":

> *Your parents are always there for you,*
> *They somehow always know what to do.*
> *If you ever have a frown*
> *You can bet they will turn it upside down.*

> *They are sweet and kind,*
> *And they always have you on their mind.*
> *Even though you may fight,*
> *They will forgive you that night.*

> *Parents are there to guide you through life,*
> *Even when you become a husband or wife.*
> *As the years pass by, keep in touch,*
> *And remember that they love you very much.*

She appeared to hit her stride at West York Senior High School, where she made a few new friends and immersed herself in her studies. A total of eight report cards covering four semesters recorded not a single mark below ninety percent, with most hovering around ninety-five to 100 percent. In Health, tenth-grade student #1250 notched a healthy ninety-seven percent.

What a difference a year makes!

The following year was even more delicious for this hungry-to-learn student. In Period 2, Semester 1, her average mark in all five subjects was a near-perfect 98.625 percent. She had achieved a goal to which she had aspired as a youngster when she predicted to her mother on October 26, 1993 — that she would "get all A's and one Not A" on her report card.

Her affinity for writing poems at age fifteen continued and began to show marked improvement. One class project was a sixteen-page book of poems that contained short and luminous pieces that provided a window into her increasingly optimistic disposition, such as this one on page three, titled "Sun."

> *Clouds swiftly opened,*
> *As the sun jumped out of them*
> *and brightened the earth.*

The booklet's title, intentionally misspelled and cryptically named *Peice of Mind in Poetry*, began with a poetic tribute to her mom, whom she still calls "adorable." Her first poem is titled "Puzzle Pieces."

> *My mom and I are like two doves,*
> *The bond we share is full of cherished moments*
> *The laughter we share brings us great joy,*
> *And the love we share is forever lasting.*

My mom and I are like puzzle pieces,
That fit perfectly together.
She's part of me.
And I'm part of her.

Valen didn't forget her father. On the next page, she typed a brief ode to her dad, on a background of a laughing, heart-shaped, single-blue-eyed Picasso-like drawing of a face with a cake and lighted candles drawn on the forehead. She called it "Icing on the Cake":

My Dad—
is the icing on a luscious piece of cake.
He makes your
eyes
twinkle with happiness,
Your
heart
open with joy,
and your
voice
ring with laughter.

By now, the young poetess was signing her name by extending the swirling "r" in "Cover" with a heart.

She continued her love of acting on school stages. She appeared in a small play called *Inside Out* for the benefit of elderly people who came to her high school to be entertained by the students and their skits. In March 2000, while attending West York High School, the young performer played the mayor's wife in the musical *Bye Bye Birdie*. Ironically, her role called for her to faint. Pam recalled, sardonically, "She did a very good job, dropping to the floor!" Later, Valen discovered she had suffered a kidney cyst bleed.

The sweet sixteen-year-old continued to flourish in her eleventh-grade academic subjects. On April 25, 2000, she was selected as a card-carrying member of the National Honor Society of Secondary Schools, which bases membership on scholarship, leadership, service, and character.

Academically, she was a rising star. Physically, her star was falling. The cysts that had taken root on her kidneys began to bleed. The cyst bleeds were painful and, in the beginning, sporadic. But they became more frequent. Despite this latest regression in her health, she did not allow it to interfere with her dream to graduate, go to college, and become a kindergarten teacher. She was determined that no bloody cyst bleeds were going to interfere with the realization of her goal. When she was just four years old, she had learned at Faith Bible Fellowship Church in York that "if thou canst believe, all things are possible to those that believeth" and, by God, she believed with all her heart that she would survive and thrive. In June, she passed with a grade point average (GPA) of 97.4 and she ranked twenty-first among the school's 186 eleventh graders.

In the summer of 2000, it was obvious the cysts on her kidneys were not going away. But the Covers were. They packed the car and headed to their favorite family vacation spot, along with Grandma Emily. The five were headed for Myrtle Beach, South Carolina.

The Grand Strand is a sixty-mile crescent of beach in this community of 25,000 permanent residents and millions of annual visitors on South Carolina's northern coast. The entire family loved the clean, wide beaches. Bill was attracted by the more than 100 golf courses along the Grand Strand, and Pam loved basking in the sun.

On the day they arrived at the Atlantic Ocean playground, misfortune struck. Valen became violently ill. It was the most serious and painful bout of cyst bleeds she had encountered thus far. She was rushed to the hospital to stem the bleeding and she remained there for a week before a decision was made to medivac her to a hospital back home, because she was too ill to travel by car. The entire cost of the flight in the emergency medical plane was borne by the company that Bill works for, Edwin L. Heim Company, an electrical, telecommunication, and mechanical construction firm in Harrisburg that was established in 1931. Bill, Brandon, and Grandma Emily made the 450-mile trek back to York in the family car while Pam accompanied her daughter in the small airplane. The agonizing four-hour flight would mark one of the last times Pam would set foot in an airplane of any kind until a trip with Bill to Mexico's Mayan Riviera in April 2008.

Once safely back in Pennsylvania, Valen was treated in the hospital for the bleeding cysts. As bad as it was, it proved to be the least of her worries. While in the hospital she developed a severe pain in the upper abdomen. Doctors soon diagnosed pancreatitis, a painful inflammation of the pancreas.

The pancreas is a large gland behind the stomach that secretes digestive enzymes into the small intestine through a tube called the pancreatic duct. These enzymes help digest fats, proteins, and carbohydrates in food. The pancreas also releases the hormones insulin and glucagon into the bloodstream. Those hormones help the body use the glucose it takes from food for energy. Normally, digestive enzymes do not become active until they reach the small intestine, where they begin digesting food. But if these enzymes become active inside the pancreas, they start "digesting" the pancreas itself.

Acute pancreatitis can be caused by gallstones or by drinking too much alcohol, but these aren't the only causes. It could have developed from pain medicine, or, as some of Valen's doctors suspected, her cyst-filled kidneys were pushing on the pancreas, causing inflammation. Treatment for acute pancreatitis can include intravenous fluids, oxygen, antibiotics, or surgery. All were considered for Valen; most were implemented. Except surgery. She was extremely ill. But the good news was that acute pancreatitis usually improves on its own with treatment designed to support vital bodily functions and the prevention of complications. Valen was kept in the hospital for several weeks while the pancreas slowly healed. In a process called total parenteral nutrition, solid food and liquids were withheld, and she was fed liquids intravenously through a feeding tube.

Valen missed fifty-eight days of school in the first two terms of her final year at high school, but in time she was well enough to return to class at West York Senior High. And return she did, with renewed determination. Where there's a will there's a way, and Valen found a way to make up for lost time. She studied like there was no tomorrow. Determined to make her parents proud, she resumed where she left off: with marks in the mid-to-high 90s. In the final four terms that year, she missed only 13.5 days of school due to illness.

The girl who was afflicted with allergies, asthma, grand mal seizures, polycystic kidney disease, scoliosis, and pancreatitis finished her last year of high school with a 95.8 GPA; her class ranking was twenty-second out of 185 students; she was one of ten students to receive a teacher-nominated Academic Achievement Award for Improvement and Effort; was named an Honoree in the York County Chamber of Commerce Honor Award Program; and was among thirty-six graduating students to receive a scholarship as part of the West York Area *Dollars for Scholars.*

Her high school days were now over. Socially, she had missed out on a lot. There had been no steady boyfriends. Her illnesses usually stood in the way of that. There were guys she had crushes on and she went to a few dances, but male friends were "buddies" who hung out in co-ed groups that she was a part of. She missed Homecoming, a rite of passage for all high school graduates. She was too ill to attend.

However, newspaper photographs of West York's graduating class of 2001 is pictorial evidence of a stunningly attractive, slim-faced, eighteen-year-old Valen with long, curly, blonde hair; eyes as bright as glowing stars; and a smile to warm the planet.

Now, it was on to college!

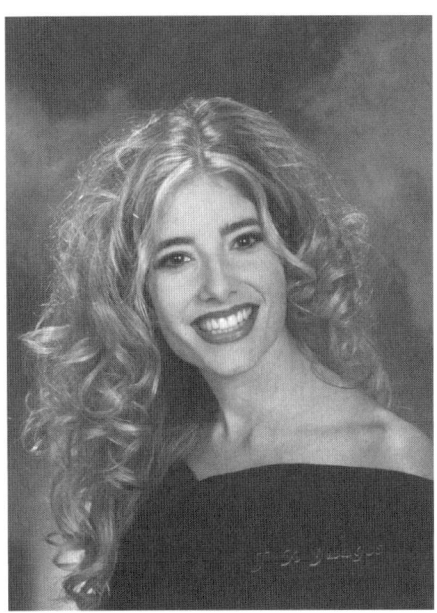

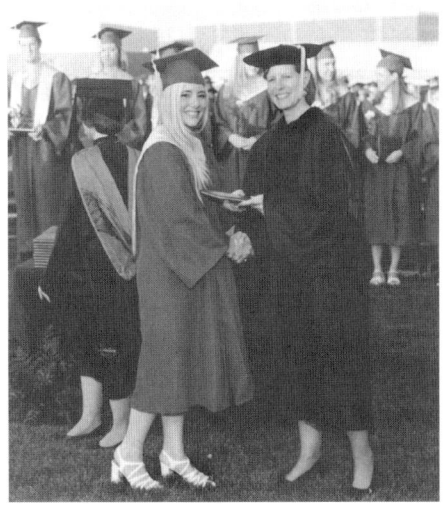

High school graduate, 2001.

Valen's high school senior year photo.

Valen had served as a kindergarten teacher's aide during her junior and senior high school years and she loved it, so the decision to pursue her dream to become a kindergarten teacher by enrolling in a place of higher learning was a no-brainer. She chose Millersville University in the small town of Millersville, Pennsylvania, idyllically situated between spacious Amish farmland and the bustling city of Lancaster.

Valen was excited about everything the next four years of college might offer, socially, creatively, and scholastically. The world was her oyster. As one of 1,300 freshmen the college admits each year, the water-loving student might read the works of American poet Henry Wadsworth Longfellow, who wrote so beautifully in "The Spanish Student": "She floats upon the river of his thoughts"; or she could join one or more of the over 100 student clubs on campus. She looked forward to hanging out at the Club de 'Ville, the non-alcoholic nightclub where she could enjoy entertainment ranging from poetry readings to the raucous sound of a local band. Or, perhaps she'd revive her student stage career and appear in a musical or drama in Dutcher Hall, home of the university's theatre.

She loved the idea of living in residence at the 'Ville, although she would surely miss the company, comfort, and care of her parents in York, just twenty miles away. Her mother was ecstatic that Valen was going to college. She saw it as a turning point in everyone's life. Brandon had left home some years before, and the empty nester mother bird was looking forward to focusing on herself and her husband, exclusively, for the first time in decades, and finding happiness in her life.

As Valen's biographer, I wanted to get a feel for the place that promised a transformation in her life, so I soaked up the atmosphere of the beautiful campus on a warm, early September afternoon in 2007. As I entered the campus, past the brown brick Millersville wall that welcomes all who enter, I was impressed by the well-maintained grounds and many low-rise buildings. A white water tower with the university's name dominates the nearby landscape. I walked past Alumni Hall and Lyte Auditorium amidst a horde of students who were walking briskly in every direction, each with a backpack slung over a shoulder. It was mid-afternoon and school had started for another year. Male and female students—mostly in their late teens—wandered to classes, some stopped off at the library, and others were making a beeline for the ball fields or the stadium. A large grouping of undergrads was hanging out at the Student Memorial Center. I stopped in front of a brown-brick building with a large, black sign with white lettering under the yellow Millersville colors. It announced that this site would be the future home of the School of Education. I felt such a pang of sadness knowing that Valen would never grace its halls.

Valen's world "came crashing down," as her mother puts it, on the evening of October 17, 2001.

Valen was taking an extra-credit evening class in an effort to gain additional credits toward her course. When the Wednesday evening class ended, she was looking forward to going out with her friends for a night of fun, away from the books. Her hair was curled and she had on one of her prettiest dresses. She left the building, skipped down a few steps, and was about to make her way to a walkway that led to her third-floor dormitory room, when a severe pain shot into her back and kidneys, causing her to stumble onto the ground. It was the most excruciating pain she had ever felt. She slowly and painfully stumbled toward her dorm room to tell her roommate and high school friend, Emily, what was happening.

When she reached the stairwell near her room, she called her doctor and said she had never before experienced such a level of pain. She vividly recalls plugging her left ear with her finger to drown out the noise of the students who were passing her on the stairs, laughing and shouting out to their friends as they scrambled out of the residence on their way to a night of fun and games. Valen remembers wanting to join them but instinctively knew she would be spending the next few hours trying to get through the night and emerge unscathed from this latest bout of pain. On the doctor's advice, she went directly to the school nurse, who administered pain medicine and ordered her to bed.

The short walk from the clinic to her residence was the longest journey she had ever taken. "I could barely make it up the one hill," she said years later, wincing at the memory. When she staggered into her room she left the door open and crawled into bed. A feeling of helplessness and hopelessness prevailed as Valen's pain persisted.

She had been in residence a mere six weeks, so she did not know a lot of people. But a male acquaintance came into the room and asked if there was anything he could do. Valen said she did not want to be alone. He stayed throughout the night, caring for her, cracking jokes to try to cheer her up, lying with her on her bed as she explained to him about PKD. He had never heard of it. He had no idea why she was in such pain. Author Naomi Wolf wrote that "pain is real when you get other people to believe in it. If no one believes in it but you, your pain is madness and hysteria."

Valen's friends knew she was in agonizing pain; they just didn't know why. Nor did she. She was just aware it had to do with her kidneys. And she was scared. "He stayed with me all night. He was so sweet. I will probably never see him again in my lifetime but I will always remember him." His name was Noah. Six years later, she would meet another Noah who would become a central figure in her life.

The next morning, she awoke bent over in pain. She immediately vomited into her white, heart-shaped trash can. Some spewed onto her pajamas. She asked her roommate to take her to the hospital. As Emily guided her friend down the stairs from their dorm, Valen took just one possession with her: her trash can. "I remember walking past my fellow students and I knew my time at Millersville University had come to an end," she revealed to me a half-dozen years later. "I knew this was different from anything I had ever experienced. Whatever was happening would change my life forever."

Her prescient knowledge was uncanny. Add "foreknowledge" to this woman's list of talents!

It took Emily just thirty minutes to deliver her friend to the emergency entrance of Milton S. Hershey Medical Center. Located in Hershey, just ten miles east of Harrisburg, the sprawling, 555-acre medical campus of Pennsylvania State University would become Valen's home for nearly two months.

The town has been synonymous with chocolate ever since Milton S. Hershey completed construction in 1905 of what would become the world's largest chocolate manufacturing plant. When I toured "the sweetest place on earth" in the summer of 2007, my taste buds were on high alert as the sweet smell of chocolate seemed to hover like a fine, invisible mist throughout the century-old Hershey Park amusement center. It saddened me to learn that Hershey is moving a big chunk of its production to Mexico.

Hershey Medical Center is without question a world-class facility with over 500 physicians on staff. Even though it is one of the nation's leading health-care establishments, with its full spectrum of advanced medical and surgical diagnostics and treatments, it could do nothing to sweeten the stay of one particular freshman college student.

Incredibly, when Valen was admitted to the hospital, she still had not informed her parents of her latest episode. "I hated to worry them and I didn't want to stress them out any more," she would say, years later. "I knew what it did to them when I had my cyst bleeds, so I tried not to involve them." Her mother admitted it was brave of her daughter to try to deal with it herself, but she conceded she and her husband were angry at Valen's "bullheadedness" when they got the call from Valen later that day. Her father couldn't suppress a feeling of pride for his only daughter. "She was away from home, growing up, going to college, and she just wanted to express her independence by handling it on her own."

But she couldn't handle it. No one could.

She was given a CT abdominal scan that Thursday, and in the sixteen days that followed, she was admitted and discharged from the hospital twice. When her friends dressed in scary and ghoulish costumes on the night of Wednesday, October 31st, Valen's hospital gown was her costume. She was discharged November 3rd, and felt well enough to return to Millersville University full of hope and dreams of the future.

But it was not to be.

At two a.m. on November 8th, Valen awoke in her dormitory bed vomiting and suffering extreme pain on her left side. Her mother went to get her. She was very, very ill. The next day, she was admitted to Hershey Medical Center once again, where her mysterious condition would confound doctors in that hospital for the next thirty-three days.

She was subjected to a battery of tests and placed on a steady diet of pain medicine. Her kidney cysts would not stop bleeding. There was blood in her urine every time she urinated. Her abdomen became bloated as the cysts filled with blood. One doctor said she looked "eleven months pregnant." Because of the blood loss, multiple transfusions were administered.

"My days at Hershey blurred into an endless time of uncontrollable pain, continuous tests, and unanswered questions," she sighed. "I developed pancreatitis again and had to be fed through a line in my arm. I couldn't stop peeing blood. I became severely exhausted, physically and mentally." The days passed relentlessly. She had little to be thankful for on Thursday, November 22, 2001, as people gobbled down Thanksgiving turkeys in households across America. Pam remembers taking Valen to the car in the hospital parking lot where they would listen to Pam's favorite rock group, Aerosmith, and its lead singer, Steven Tyler. Pam found Tyler "mesmerizing and incredibly sexy" and she admitted that she relates to some of the band's hit songs, like "Dream On" and "Fly Away from Here." "Those songs would make me drift off to a comfortable, peaceful, soulful place," she wrote to me in October 2007. "I still smile when I hear those songs on the radio."

Doctors and nurses at Hershey could not disguise their dismay regarding the difficult case. They were perplexed that Valen was not responding to treatment. And the parents and patient were becoming despondent. Everyone shared a common concern: she might not survive. Pam was familiar with the English proverb, "While the doctors consult, the patient dies," but if she had anything to do with it, there was no way in hell she would sit idly by while her second-born went to an early grave.

More than a month after Valen was last admitted to Hershey, there was no obvious sign of relief in sight, and hope was quickly fading for a recovery anytime soon. Pam set the wheels in motion to have Valen transferred to another hospital. Call it grasping at straws or in search of a miracle; it really was a last-ditch effort to save her child. Valen's resourceful and determined mother made countless phone calls, waded through a mountain of research, and with assistance from the Hershey staff, corresponded with a legion of medical experts.

Her diligence paid off.

She met Dr. Terry Watnick of the Division of Nephrology at Johns Hopkins School of Medicine, 720 Rutland Avenue, Baltimore, Maryland, whose tiny office on the ninth floor of the Ross Building would become a portal to a ray of light that would eventually shine upon Pam's sick daughter.

4

The Johns Hopkins Adventure

"When there is pain, there are no words.
All pain is the same."
—*Toni Morrison*

To merely suggest that Johns Hopkins is a historic name in medicine is an understatement of monumental proportion.

The famed Baltimore institution uses the all-encompassing name Johns Hopkins Medicine to identify its hospital and health system and its school of medicine. It is widely regarded as one of the world's greatest hospitals. When Johns Hopkins, a Quaker merchant, banker, and businessman, left seven million dollars in 1873 to create a university and hospital, he could not have foreseen that it would become a four-billion-dollar organization with bricks and mortar totaling 4.2 million square feet where 25,949 people work together to help save lives and discover cures and wash windows and pay accounts receivable and teach medical students and hold the hands of terrified teenagers with bleeding kidney cysts. Today, The Johns Hopkins Hospital and University is the state's largest private employer.

The establishment unites the physicians and scientists of the Johns Hopkins University School of Medicine with the health professionals and facilities that make up the broad Johns Hopkins Health System. It is a formidable institution by any standard. The university boasts a former president as one of its graduates (Woodrow Wilson, Ph.D. 1886, History), and nineteen current or former School of Medicine scientists are Nobel Prize winners, including Wilson's Nobel Peace Prize in 1919. Thirty-two Nobel Prize winners have had an association at some point in time with The Johns Hopkins University, either as graduates or as faculty.

On the frosty day of Tuesday, December 11, 2001, Valen Cover became one of 47,378 annual admissions to Johns Hopkins Hospital. She was placed in one of the 1,017 patient beds in a building that would become her home for the next 105 days.

Bill and Pam began to walk the halls of the world-famous institution with a sense of cautious optimism. They knew of the stellar international reputation of the Johns Hopkins Hospital — or JH, as it's known locally — and that it has been ranked the number one hospital in the United States every year since 1992 by *U.S. News & World Report;* that its 1,714 attending physicians, 1,089 residents and fellows, and 8,817 employees working in twenty interconnected buildings were among the cream of the crop in the country's health care system.

But could their combined efforts help their daughter?

Dr. Terry Watnick, a graduate of Yale Medical School and Assistant Professor of Medicine in the Division of Nephrology was the first expert at JH to attempt to answer the question.

A slight woman in her late forties with an effervescent smile and long, thick, brunette hair accented with large, oval glasses in a silver frame, Dr. Watnick has an enviable track record of notable accomplishments in the PKD field. She has headed the hospital's Hereditary Renal Disease Clinic and was instrumental in developing the methods that now form the basis for the only commercially available DNA

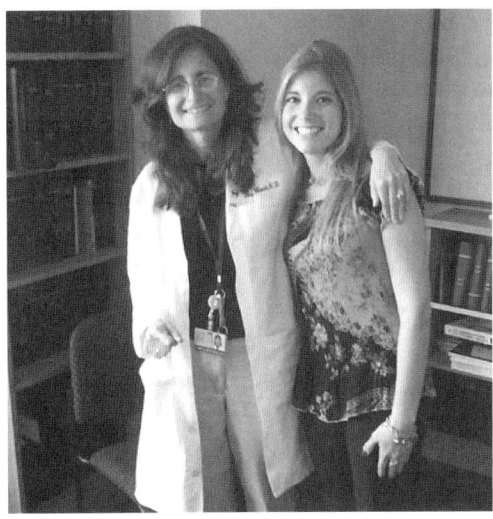

Valen visited Dr. Terry Watnick in the nephrologist's office in 2007.

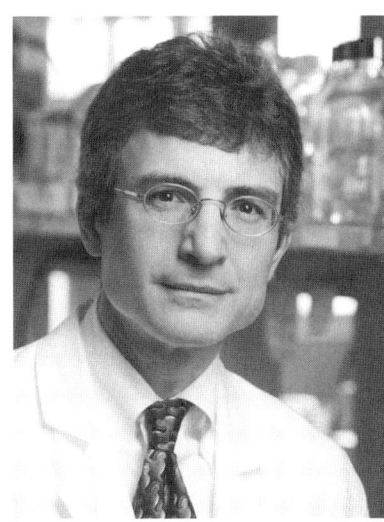

Dr. Gregory Germino.

test for PKD1, one of the two genes that cause ADPKD, the kind that appeared to be slowly killing Valen. She works closely with her husband, Dr. Gregory G. Germino, Professor of Medicine in the Division of Nephrology and Professor in the Department of Molecular Biology and Genetics. The couple has four children. In the summer of 2002, Dr. Germino and teams of researchers, working independently at the Mayo Clinic and Johns Hopkins University, isolated the gene responsible for autosomal recessive polycystic kidney disease (ARPKD) and traced its mode of expression.

Dr. Watnick has taken care of a lot of PKD patients throughout her career, but Valen's was a problem she had rarely encountered. Normally, people with PKD can expect their cysts to burst and bleed. In the vast majority of cases, it is self-limited, and with some bedrest, the bleeding stops in about three days. But in Valen's case, they bled and bled, continually. She received scores of blood transfusions but the cause of the persistent bleeding was a mystery. Dr. Watnick was the attending physician and she told me that she "agonized" over Valen's case. One choice was to remove the football-size kidneys, but Valen was young and her kidney function at that time was relatively good despite their abnormal size. Besides, there was no donor waiting in the wings. Her father's blood was not a match and her mother and brother and most of Pam's family have PKD. Dr. Watnick and the Covers knew the statistics as well as anyone: approximately 70,000 people were waiting for a kidney transplant in the United States; the wait averages about five years, during which time 30,000 will either die or become too sick for a transplant.

When all attempts to block off the recurrent bleeding with injections and embolization proved fruitless, Dr. Watnick called in the experts. She consulted with many, including Dr. Mark Hughes,

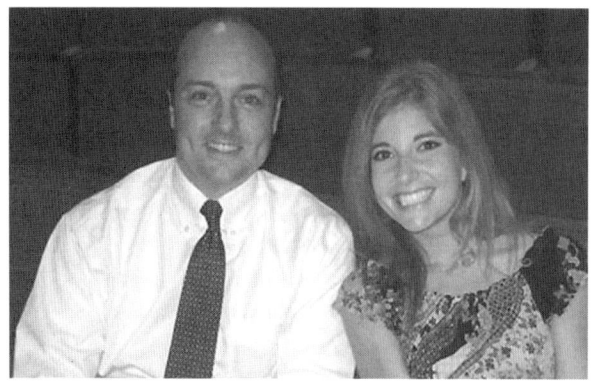

Valen's internist at Johns Hopkins, Dr. Mark Hughes, knew at age four that he wanted to become a doctor.

the brilliant Assistant Professor of Medicine in the Division of General Internal Medicine at the Johns Hopkins University School of Medicine. Among his impressive research and teaching credentials, his professional interests include advance care planning, end-of-life decision-making, and ethics consultation.

When I met with the forty-one-year-old doctor at 9:00 a.m. on Friday, August 31, 2007, in the Schaeffer Auditorium on the fourth floor of the Children's Medical Center at JH, we talked about his dream at age four of becoming a doctor. "My great-aunt gave me a real stethoscope—not a toy one—so that solidified it for me then and there," he said, smiling as dimples deepened in his young-looking face. We met to discuss what he called "Valen's triumph over adversity," but he admitted when he first treated the seriously ill teenager, hers was one of the more complex cases he had seen. "It was a very complicated case, and few institutions I know of, other than Johns Hopkins, could have handled this kind of complexity because of the different levels of specialization required to address all of the issues," he said, adding that Hershey Medical Center is a fine institution but even it regarded Valen's case as too complex for them to handle.

The difficulty arose in part because so many of Valen's organs and bodily systems were involved. As soon as one problem was corrected, another would arise. She was on multiple medications and was becoming a habitual resident in the intensive care unit (ICU), where she was often placed on a ventilator. Add to that, she was becoming demoralized at being so chronically ill for so long.

An endless variety of tests was being administered to no avail, and December 25th was just another day in a hospital ward for Valen. There would be no letters to Santa from brother Brandon, saying: "Valen and I have been pretty bad this year, but still try to give us a couple of presents." Bill and Pam decorated Valen's room to make it Christmassy and gave her presents, including costume jewelry, but the only gift Valen wanted this Christmas was a healthy body.

As Valen's internist, Dr. Hughes saw his role as attending to all the multiple medical issues and orchestrating the specialists. And he had a lot of leading physicians to call upon. In addition to Valen's nephrologist, Dr. Watnick, there was a gastroenterologist to deal with the pancreas problem, and a neurologist to treat her "morbidly elevated" high blood pressure. Urologists Dr. Thomas Jarrett and

Dr. Ronald Rodriguez were an integral part of the process to determine, "Where do we go from here in the long term?"

The primary strategy was to stop the bleeding from her right, irritated, and inflamed kidney. Intervention radiology procedures were conducted to try and isolate the cysts and stop the bleeding, but when that failed, there were ongoing discussions about removing just her right, bleeding kidney. Then the left kidney started to bleed, and doctors were faced with the fact that the bleeds could be ongoing, indefinitely, until she died. They were aware of the intense pain she was enduring, which the numerous narcotics could not dull and antibiotics could not cure. The case was considered multifactorial and multifarious. Two big words for a little person in such dire straits.

As the medical experts conferred and treated Valen, her condition was becoming grave. Dr. Watnick agonized over removing the kidneys of such a young person, never forgetting that the waiting period for a new, donated kidney could be up to five years, depending on the blood type. "That's a long time for anyone to be on dialysis," she remarked to me.

Bill and Pam were always an integral part of all discussions, as was Valen, to the best of her ability. When it was decided to remove the kidneys, Dr. Hughes referred to it as a "substantial decision and a seminal moment." With the judgment call made, the medical team lost no time in calling in Dr. Robert A. Montgomery, one of the world's leading kidney transplant surgeons and director of Hopkins' transplant center. They wanted Dr. Montgomery's involvement due to the complexity of the surgery required on such enlarged kidneys. And if a donor kidney were found, could the surgery be performed soon, so she would not be on dialysis for a long period of time?

It was determined that a bilateral nephrectomy (surgical removal of left and right kidneys) would be performed in a procedure that would have "limited morbidity." At the time, Dr. Jarrett (now Urology Chair at George Washington University) was one of the few urologists performing laparoscopic procedures, and it was hoped that a small incision could enable the surgeon to get at the kidneys and remove them. There was little optimism in the procedure—considering the size of Valen's kidneys—but with input from the parents, the patient, and the medical people involved, and with seemingly no other viable options, they gave it a try.

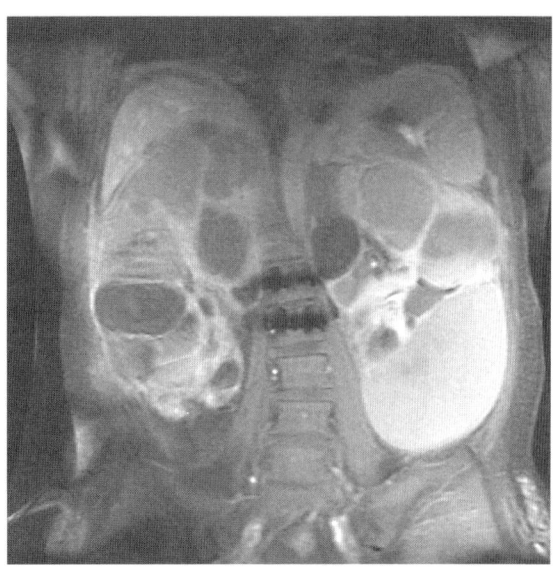

View of Valen's football-sized kidneys prior to their removal.

On January 25, 2002 — eleven days before her nineteenth birthday — both of Valen's massive, cyst-filled kidneys were removed.

"And that's when all the crap started," says Valen.

When she awoke from the bilateral nephrectomy, she had a 15.5-inch scar that stretched under her rib cage; painful pancreatitis; and a catheter in her arm to support the blood-cleansing dialysis sessions that she would endure immediately.

She was facing an uncertain future.

During the daily dialysis sessions that followed, she wondered if and when a kidney would become available. "I hit my lowest point ever, after the surgery," she confided to me years later.

By February 4th, she was back in the ICU, because she was vomiting blood clots and there was blood in her stool. It took several endoscopic procedures over the next few days before doctors were able to determine that the source of the blood was a bleeding vessel and four bleeding ulcers in her stomach. She lost such a vast amount of blood, she was fed eleven units of blood intravenously — in one day.

But it wasn't enough to compensate for the large amount of lost blood. Just two weeks following her bilateral nephrectomy, Valen required emergency surgery to repair her damaged stomach. Prior to the surgery, more expert opinions were sought and there was talk of removing her stomach. There ensued a round of discussions, consultations, debates, and deliberations by some of the finest medical minds in the country. The ultimate decision was made by

Dr. Pamela A. Lipsett, currently Professor of Surgery, ACCM and Nursing Surgical Critical Care Fellowship Director in the Department of Surgery & Surgical Sciences at Johns Hopkins Medicine: Every effort would be made to save the girl's stomach.

"The Death Watch." That's how Valen refers to the afternoon before her stomach surgery. Her family and friends were advised to visit before the operation because doctors were uncertain if her ravaged body could handle another traumatic procedure. Valen sensed a strange and unsettling feeling of morbidity on this particular afternoon. "We had to put the game face on," her father revealed to me several years later. "We never, ever misled her, but sometimes it was horrible to watch. There were times she did not look like a human being."

She considered it strange seeing her mother, father, brother, Brandon, and close family and friends all gathered in one ICU room—and all at the same time. Brandon was running his own small business in York and helping to care for his newborn son, so he was not able to visit his sister often in the Baltimore hospital. When she saw him to her left in the cramped room, she knew the prognosis was grave.

She lay in the antiseptic hospital bed under a white, starched linen sheet that felt like a shroud, and she gazed into everyone's eyes, struggling to remain calm as worried thoughts thundered in her brain. A macabre silence filled the room. A family friend, Dick Mansberger, who works with her father, stood by her bed holding her frail hand. She spoke not a word. "Mom was sitting on a chair to my right. The look on her face told me things were definitely not good. Dad stood next to me, a look of helplessness etched on his handsome face. I was fearful, but I stayed focused and I refused to allow doubt to enter my mind. I said nothing. Not a single word to anyone. I was determined to live through this. I would have plenty of time to talk later."

She was right. The operation was a success. Her bone-weary body had now been subjected to over seventy blood transfusions. She was drained, emotionally and physically. She was weak and dead tired. But she was alive and thankful for that!

The agonizing days, weeks, and months that followed proved to be a slow but steady climb toward recovery. And she knows she would not have made it without the love and support of two very special people.

5

The Parents

Parents decide to accept the responsibility of raising children.
Any thanks they get for doing that is gravy. Grateful children
are a blessing . . . but they aren't a necessity."
— *From the book* Children under Stress *(1983)*

The above words were written the year Valen Cover was born, and if anyone can show me a child more grateful for the love of two people on this earth, well, that's more bubblegum than I can chew.

In the few years I have known Valen, I have admired in her what writer Thomas Gray calls "the still small voice of gratitude." It's a joyful thing to be thanked, and Valen appreciates and acknowledges the goodness and thoughtfulness of everyone who is kind to her. She has thanked me for things as simple as phoning her for no particular reason; for treating her to a Caramel Frappuccino at Starbucks; sending her inspirational books and cards; a hammock Kris and I purchased for her rented farmhouse; and for a billion gazillion other seemingly innocuous things. Her sincerity is genuine and her attitude is modest and demure. But when it comes to expressing gratitude to her parents for all they have done, she would—if she could—shout it out from the top of the beautiful Victorian dome of the Johns Hopkins Hospital Building that has been a landmark of the Baltimore skyline since 1889.

Bill and Pam were born in the same delivery room in 1956 in York Hospital, just 104 days apart. Evelyn B. Snyder, R.N., signed both birth certificates. It wasn't until the early spring of 1976 that the pretty, long-haired, twenty-year-old, who showed a flair for art and creative writing in high school, met her handsome and popular future husband. Like Pam, Bill was also raised in York. He had played a little football and basketball in junior high school and excelled in baseball and golf in senior high. Their first encounter was at a bowling alley, one of the favorite hangout spots for York's youth in those days. They were married at seven p.m. on August 14, 1976, and wasted no time starting a family. "Bill was so cute, and we were madly in love," Pam confided to me after their thirty-first wedding anniversary. "But it was not a match made in heaven."

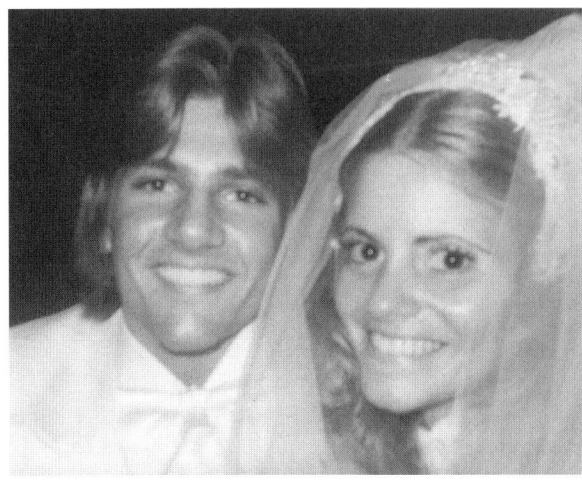

Bill and Pam's wedding day.

The couple separated when Brandon was three years old. "We separated twice," Pam admitted. "When we got back together the second time, I told Bill we were meant for each other. I waited for his comment and commitment, and he said: 'No, Pam, I don't think so. We have to work at it.' He was being honest. Communication is so important."

I spent an evening with them in their cozy home on York's Susquehanna Trail in late summer 2007. It was an unforgettable four hours. I wanted to know as much as I could about Valen's parents. We started with some family background.

Bill's father, William, was suffering from advanced Alzheimer's disease when he died in 2003. Bill's mother, Emily Elizabeth, is an active octogenarian who walks her dog sometimes four times a day near her home in nearby Fireside, where Bill grew up. His sister, Joanne, seven years Bill's junior, also lives in the area. Together with her husband, Rick, and their two sons, Ricky and Ryan, the couple hosts an annual family picnic that is notable as much for the fresh grilled venison, corn on the cob, and other fixings, as it is for the kegs of fresh, cold, pour-it-yourself Yuengling Lager. I speak as one who feasted and imbibed at the 3rd annual outdoor summer fest!

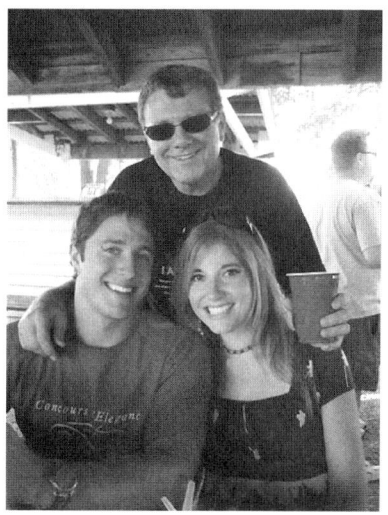

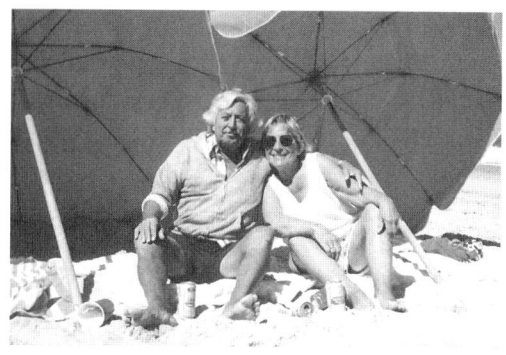

Bill's parents, Emily and William Cover, at the beach.

Dennis joins Valen's boyfriend, Noah, and Valen at an annual family picnic in August 2007.

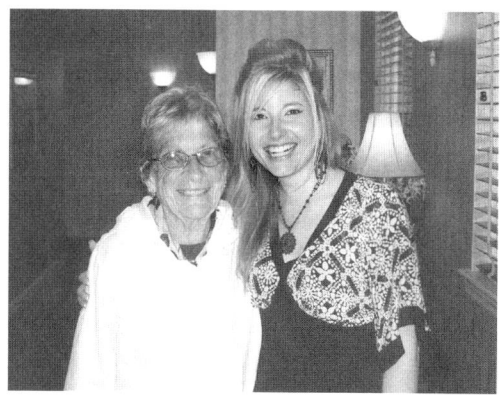

Grandma Emily and granddaughter Valen.

From fifth grade on, Pam grew up in the Susquehanna Trail home with her mother, Pauline, who was known as "Mickey," and stepfather, Spike. Her birth father died while she was in senior high school. PKD claimed the life of her mother on November 7, 1981, at age fifty-three, after being on dialysis for seven years. When Pam's sister, Donna Marie Feather, died in 1999, Spike promised Pam she could

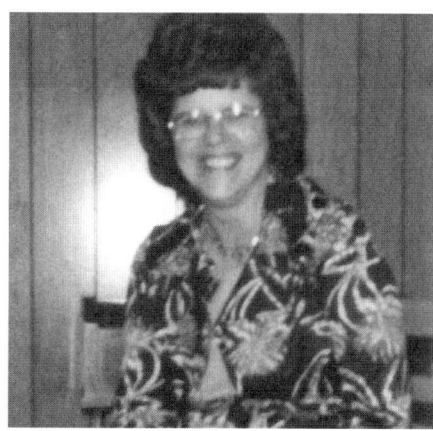

Pam's mother, Pauline.

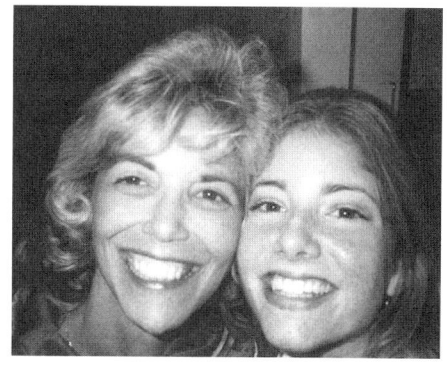

Valen and Aunt Donna the summer before Donna passed away, a victim of PKD.

have the house when he passed on. When Spike died on July 9, 2000, the four Covers were living in the large home in West York. Later, when Valen became very sick and her parents were hit with huge medical bills, Pam said the promise of the house was a godsend. "There was no way we could have kept up with the mortgage payments and dealt with Valen's bills at the same time," she revealed.

Today, Pam calls her daughter "our little miracle," and it's obvious she dotes on her—from filling out her medical insurance forms, to taking her shopping for clothes at Kohl's Department Store, armed with thirty-percent-off coupons.

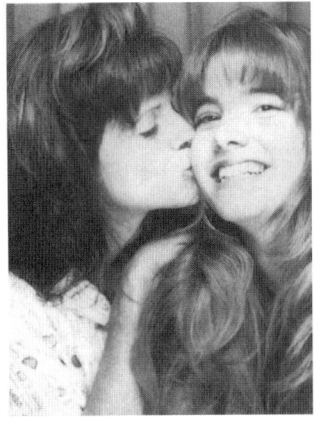
Valen and her mom drop into a picture booth after seeing a movie.

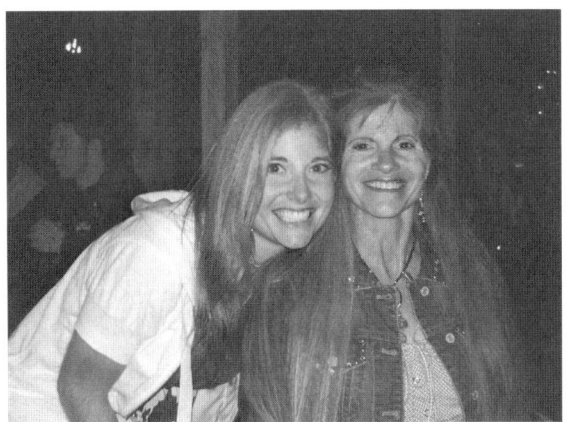
Mom and daughter enjoying a night out at T.J. Rockwell's American Grill & Tavern with friends and family, summer 2007.

One of Pam's greatest passions in life is her love of all animals, especially horses.

"Animals over most people," Bill murmured.

"Absolutely," Pam agreed, promptly. "Animals are not judgmental. They are not critical. They love and appreciate the care and attention they receive."

For the past several years, Pam has volunteered her time at a local 200-acre farm owned by Eugene "Gene" Garrod, owner of Garrod Hydraulics. He founded the company in 1978 and grew it to be the largest industrial hard-chrome-plating shop on the East Coast. Pam's labor-of-love chores include feeding horses, mowing, and beautifying the property with flowers in the summer and Christmas decorations in the winter. In spring, Pam uses a John Deere tractor to pull a heavily built rotary mower—called a brush hog—to mow the pastures and horse trail that surround the acreage. She also climbs aboard a Kabota Zero-Turn riding mower to mow areas around barns, yards, and laneways. By mid-to-late summer, she can be found stacking hay in the barn to prepare for the coming winter. She "drags" various pastures with a John Deere tractor and a smaller Gator, checks water containers, sweeps the barns, and performs plenty of other chores, because, as she says, "There's always something to do on a farm."

Bill tolerates his wife's hobby, suggesting she has earned this time for herself. "She was dedicated to raising her family and never really had time for hobbies, and now she does, and that's a good thing. And look at those muscles!" He didn't have to draw attention to Pam's muscle-bound upper arms, because I witnessed her powerful physique in action three months earlier when I spent a morning with her and watched in awe as she hefted heavy bales of hay like they were pounds of butter.

When I first divulged to Pam that I would be writing her daughter's life story, I explained that I would be seeking background information that only she would be aware of and could reveal. Her reply was honest and forthright. "I have put memories in chests and drawers behind locked doors down a long, long hallway. I have chosen to put some things away in a safe place in my mind so I can fill it with new things. I have not gone down that hallway for a long time and have surely not opened some of those doors for awhile." She also acknowledged, a little warily, that her daughter, too, would have to "dig down deep into her darkest days and explore her darkest feelings to express what she has been through." Her response unnerved me slightly. From the outset, Valen predicted that her mother would be "the key" to providing long-forgotten details for the book. What if she wouldn't cooperate?

Pam is a very thoughtful person who will pause inscrutably before responding to a question or remark. She abhors small talk, possesses a highly honed bullshit detector, and does not suffer fools gladly. I recognized those qualities during our second rendezvous (the first was in a pub with family and friends), when she and I met for an early morning cheese omelet breakfast at York's 'Round the Clock Diner. I must have been desperate to impress her, because I blabbered on about how her daughter has the potential, ability, and smarts to accomplish any dream to which she aspires, and that Valen should not aim for the moon when she can reach the stars and blah blah blah. I soon realized that the horse lover sitting opposite me in her favorite Levi jeans and a form-fitting T-shirt with HOWDY written across her chest was making polite hand gestures that indicated I was piling the bullshit higher and deeper. I knew right then we would become good friends, and we have. Pam reassured me that it would take time to reveal to me what is in those chests and drawers. When she dropped me off at the Harrisburg airport later that day for my return trip to Toronto, she hopped out of the farm truck, hugged me, and said: "Thank you, Dennis, for taking Valen into your heart." She placed her hand over her heart. "It means a lot to us."

Since that airport hug on May 9, 2007, scores of e-mails and phone calls have been shared between us. She has sent me a treasure trove of material on a smorgasbord of topics, from what she was making for dinner on a particular evening, to how she likes to decorate Gene's barn at Christmas with garlands and bright lights. And she related funny stories about Valen as a child. Here's just one: "When Valen was three years old, she was a very inquisitive child. Whenever I was on the phone she was a 'sticky boogy.' She made it appear that she was doing her own thing but she was listening to every word I was saying on the phone. Sometimes, when the other party hung up, I would stay on the line and say: 'Yes, uh-huh, I have a daughter. Yes, she is three . . . yes, she's for sale . . . no, she's pretty cheap — in fact she's free.' Valen would stop what she was doing and I had so much fun seeing her reaction. Oh, she was so cute and she knew that I loved her dearly and she also knew in her heart this was not at all true."

While Pam excelled at art and creative writing in school, she had no formal writing training; yet her many mini-essays to me (some e-mails exceed 1,500 words) are filled with the kind of description and characterization that is taught at university creative writing classes. In one letter, she revealed that Valen had a crush on a "large, handsome, broad-shouldered, black-haired doctor who wore a long white jacket when he checked on Valen. As soon as he'd leave the room, Valen would make a sound like she just ate a wonderful dessert."

One day, Valen and her mom were walking around the hospital ward for exercise. Valen was wearing shorts. When the handsome doctor passed by, Pam and Valen said his eyes went "from Valen's face, down her body and back up." Afterwards, they were like two excited school girls with overactive hormones. "Oh my gosh, Mom," Valen exclaimed. "He checked me out!" Pam said her daughter's ear-to-ear smile was priceless and precious. Pam admitted that she, too, had a school-girl type of crush on a different doctor, and when Valen asked him one day what kind of car he drove, he answered: "An Audi." Pam suppressed a mischievous giggle and wanted to say, but didn't: "She asked what kind of car you drive, not what kind of belly button you have!" (Get it? An "outi.") One day, just before the same doctor entered the room on his rounds, Pam, in her boredom, had cut slits around the edges of her own yellow, mandatory hospital smock, to make a sexier version of her gown.

In a lengthy e-mail to me in November 2007, Pam bared her soul about her marriage difficulties during the peak of Valen's illness at Johns Hopkins, conceding that the days, weeks, and months took a toll on her and Bill. Others noticed the tension. A doctor asked if she had considered killing herself; and a nurse suggested they take turns caring for their daughter to relieve the stress and pressure. "This was a very low point in our relationship," she confided. "We had no one to lean on when things got really tough. I could not comfort him and he could not comfort me, because we expended all our energy comforting Valen."

Pam was forthright when she said a new partner for both of them might have been the answer, but she explained her decision to stick it out by comparing a new husband to her makeup mirror. Her reasoning was enlightening: "I bought my original makeup mirror at a supermarket thirty years ago. Over the years, I lost a cover to one of the side lights. I never once had to change a light bulb in the makeup mirror. It always did the job. Recently, I thought it was time to buy another makeup mirror, only because the other one was old. I bought a new one and threw out the old one. Not long after I discarded the old one, I realized the new one does not have an outlet to plug in a curling iron or a hair dryer as my old one did. I miss that important option. My new one makes a continuous, loud, humming noise. My old one never made a peep. My new one has side mirrors. I thought it would be nice to be able to look at my makeup from a side view. I never use it. The lights on my old one were bright. The new one is not as bright. This is what I would think if I were to change husbands: I would miss the old 'model.' Also, I believe in the vows 'for better or for worse.'"

Bill's and Pam's marriage vows had been tested very early in their marriage. Just two years after their wedding, the couple was living apart. It was an amicable separation; they dated other people but saw each other as well, in the hope of sometime getting back together.

Pam's mother, Pauline, was seriously ill with PKD. After spending so many agonizing years of dialysis, her death in November 1981 was very hard on Pam. "Bill was very kind," she told me recently. "He often came with me to visit my mother when she was in the hospital, and he accompanied me and my sister as we chose a casket. I was thankful for his presence." After the funeral, Bill and Pam talked about trying to save their marriage despite both of their admissions that the love they once felt for each other was not as deep or strong as it had been. Nevertheless, they worked at it, and in early May 1982, Pam learned she was pregnant with her second child. "I was totally surprised and happy but Bill did not take the news well," she disclosed to me. "My mother had just died from PKD six months earlier, and I had the disease. Neither of us wanted to pass this terrible condition on to another child."

Pam's gynecologist suggested she get an abortion. Pam knew that abortions were illegal at the time but her doctor assured her that this would be considered a "medical necessity" and would be approved. Pam made an appointment to terminate her pregnancy.

However, in the brief period before the scheduled date, Pam could not "come to grips" with the feeling that having an abortion was the right decision. One day, while taking a walk near her apartment, Pam spotted a woman pushing a little girl in a carriage along the sidewalk. Pam described to me the intercessional event that unfolded: "I stared at the little girl in the carriage. The woman—I assume it was her mother—never looked at me, but the little girl continued to glare at me with a penetrating look. They were across the street from me, but as I passed by, the little girl and I continued to stare at each other, not breaking eye contact for one second. I knew immediately those beautiful little eyes were telling me to have this baby inside me."

The night before Pam's appointment, she read the bible for further guidance and to "shed some light" on her situation. The next day, Bill drove her to York Hospital where the procedure would take place. They sat in the car in the parking lot for a long time, talking.

Finally, Bill said: "You don't have to have this abortion if you don't want to."

That's all Pam needed to hear. "I was so happy and relieved."

A quarter century later, they say they are thankful "for making the right decision."

Pam related the near-abortion story to me and Kris in August 2007 by a lake near York. It was a warm and bright sunny day, but Pam took a figurative walk down one of the long, dark hallways of suppressed memories she had warned me about months earlier. As she stood near the water, her long, reddish-brown hair blowing in the slight summer breeze, Pam unlocked a symbolic door and dug deep into a chest of drawers that had guarded a secret from nearly everyone—including Valen—for twenty-five years. Pam had kept the memory in an imaginary diary that she always carried with her.

On Friday, December 28, 2007, Pam invited Valen to spend the afternoon with her. Pam made lunch and they scoured through old family albums to choose photographs for this intimate biography. Pam saw it as the perfect time and opportunity to reveal her secret to the daughter she loved so much and to relieve herself of the burden and pain of this truth that had been concealed for so long.

She worried how Valen would take it. That same Friday night, I received an e-mail from Pam. "Valen has been told," she wrote. "She took it very well. We should never underestimate the power of Valen!"

A day later, I asked Valen if she would care to share her thoughts with me about learning of the near-abortion. When she agreed, I came right to the point: "What was your reaction when you learned for the first time yesterday that your mother, who was pregnant with you in 1982, had made an appointment to terminate the pregnancy and cancelled it practically at the last minute?"

Valen's response was powerful. She displayed characteristic maturity, understanding, sympathy, grace, and kindness: "After everything I have gone through in my life, not much fazes me, but I am happy Mom told me about the near-abortion. It allowed me the opportunity to learn more about her. I admire her even more now, if that's possible, for being so strong and for sacrificing so much for me. She has gone through so much pain because of me—even before I was born! I don't know how I can ever repay her or thank her for all the pain and heartache I have caused. I'm just so happy to be alive! I was more intrigued than saddened by what she revealed to me. The only thing that saddened me was imagining everything that my mom was going through at the time. Her own mother had just died from PKD; she and her dad were trying to mend their relationship; and then she finds herself pregnant again and did not want to pass on the disease to another child. It is ironic that they did not want to pass on PKD to me, yet they decided to have me, and we went through so much *because* of PKD!

"Mom was worried how I would take the news after all these years. I cried when she told me about the little girl in the stroller and how they kept staring at each other. It shows the power that one individual can have on another, because Mom pretty much decided at that moment not to go through with the abortion. I call it a miracle, and both Mom and I believe that little girl was an angel sent by God. I'm not really surprised that my life started that way, because it seems like my life has been a constant battle. I am always fighting death—in the womb; through my sicknesses; the motorcycle accident. I have been near death so many times. I wonder why I have had so many close calls. I think that's why I am somewhat impatient and I want to do so many things with my life, now."

Today, Valen is alive and breathing, as she likes to put it, and Bill and Pam are united strongly in marriage. The couple enjoys many similar—and some separate—pastimes. If Pam's obsession is working with four-legged animals, Bill's mania is reserved for golf and two-wheeled, motorized machines. York is home to a 1.5-million-square-foot Harley-Davidson plant that sits on 230 acres and employs over 3,200 people. "When I was younger, my mother would not let me have a motorcycle," he said, feigning sadness. "I went through therapy on that. Twelve-ounce therapy," he joked. When their son, Brandon, was old enough, he bought himself a 1964 Triumph chopper that needed some work. Bill visited Brandon a few times a week in nearby Red Lion, tinkered with the bike, and started to enjoy "messing around with it." So much so that Bill bought his own vintage bike in 2002, a 1967 Triumph. He enjoyed working on it after work in the shed behind the house and would be there until eleven p.m. most nights. He liked that it was something he could share with his son. Bill currently has three motorcycles: the '67 Triumph; a 1978 Triumph; and a 2003 Harley-Davidson 100th Anniversary

Road King that he bought new. Naturally, the anniversary bike was made in York.

Bill and Pam may have had their ups and downs in their married life, but they are resilient people and they weathered the storms. In late 2007, Valen said she had never seen her parents happier.

But in 2002, their daughter's spirit and body were broken, and all of Pam's horses and all of Bill's bikes couldn't put her back together again. So they did what any parent would do: they devoted all of their energy, love, and support to the survival of their daughter and to making her whole again. Pam had been by her daughter's side throughout the hospital stays and now it was time for her to move, temporarily, to Baltimore. She took a room in Maryland's only Ronald McDonald House (RMH) at 635 West Lexington Street so she could be with her daughter night and day. As the breadwinner of the family, Bill remained in his job "to keep the family afloat," as Pam put it, and to retain medical benefits.

At the beginning, the arrangement was manageable. Bill worked during the week in Harrisburg and stayed alone in the family's York home. He would join Pam to help care for their daughter every weekend and on holidays, including Christmas and New Year's. But nothing could have prepared them for the maelstrom that would sweep over them in the days and weeks that followed.

From the day Valen was admitted to Johns Hopkins, her condition worsened to the extent that her very existence was soon in question. Pam attempted to handle things by herself with part-time help from her beleaguered husband, whose heart was in Baltimore, but his mind and body in Harrisburg and York.

A nurse at the hospital took Pam aside one day and told her that her demeanor was harmful to Valen's well-being. "You need to put on a happy face to bring some sort of brightness to Valen's grim condition," the well-meaning nurse scolded. Pam felt she could not put on an act. "I was scared and worried," she confided to me years later. "I knew I was no longer supportive to Valen, as I for some reason felt that her very existence was on my shoulders."

Author William Ellery Channing wrote that difficulties are meant to rouse, not discourage. "The human spirit is to grow strong by conflict." Pam's spirit was not growing stronger. Each day seemed to bring more emotional trauma than the previous. The mental anguish of seeing her daughter in such pain was becoming unbearable. Her stress level was at an all-time high and she was near the breaking point. Soon, it was too much to bear. On a day in early January, she could take no more. Pam snapped. She was a broken woman, filled with despair and hopelessness.

In this, her darkest hour to date, Pam found herself alone and walking slowly through a corridor of the Hopkins' Billings Administration Building. Her heart was heavy with the fear that Valen would not recover. She spotted three old, cherry-colored, wooden phone booths, standing side by side. She entered one, closed the door, sat on a wooden swivel chair, and dissolved into tears. After crying her heart out, she wiped away a few remaining tears, and lifted the black phone handle from its cradle. She called her husband. "Bill, I can't do this alone anymore," was all she could blurt out between her sobs.

She slowly raised herself up, clutched the brass handle, opened the bi-fold door, and re-entered the narrow hallway. She turned right and walked the short distance to the lobby below the grand dome of the Hopkins building. She stood in front of the world-renowned, ten-and-a-half-foot statue of Jesus. The towering, marble figure depicted a calm-looking man, head bowed, and arms extended as though he were reaching out to Pam. She looked up into his eyes and spoke silently. "I put all my trust and faith in you, Jesus. I have no strength left."

The six-ton statue, called *Christus Consolator*, was erected in 1896 and has been a source of inspiration and consolation for untold numbers of patients, doctors, nurses, students, and visitors from all over the world. A replica of an 1820 work by Danish sculptor Bertel Thorvaldsen, the statue was carved from a single block of Carrara marble. It was pulled from the Baltimore harbor on a wooden sled drawn by four horses all the way up Broadway to the hospital's north entrance, and then slid down a short corridor to its present position. Since then, it has become a symbol of compassion and prayerful hope for many. Visitors and Hopkins employees alike rub the toes of the statue as they pass by, and some stop to pray in silence.

As Pam stood in the rotunda area before the statue, whispering her prayer of release, she took a deep breath. A sense of calm swept through her. "I was at the lowest point of my life," she confessed to me several years later. "I was indeed humbled. And after placing my trust in Him, I was—and still am—eternally grateful."

She felt a renewed sense of relief that day and a belief that things were going to be okay. She was overcome with a sense of peace, and she felt an emotional charge — an unexplained sensation — that she was not alone in this struggle. It was a very welcome epiphany. Five years later, Pam would return to the same phone booth with her daughter at one of the lowest times in Valen's existence, and once again a life-altering change would take place in one of the "Cover Girls" under the magnificent Johns Hopkins Dome.

Bill asked for and received a leave of absence from his management position at Edwin L. Heim Company. They paid his full salary and benefits. He joined Pam on January 15th, 2002, and for the next two and a half months, their home away from home was a bedroom on an upper floor of Ronald McDonald House.

In August 2007, Valen wanted to see, for the first time, the place from which her parents travelled four miles every day through Baltimore's busy downtown streets to stay with her until late at night.

I accompanied Valen to the house that has served as an oasis since its opening in June 1982 to 35,000 families who have needed a place to stay while their world turned upside down, as they tried to cope with the emotional and financial trauma of dealing with a deathly ill loved one. Each year, 1,500 families arrive at the doorstep of what becomes their second home for days, weeks, or months. Families pay up to fifteen dollars a night. Bill and Pam were one of thirty-six families who occupied rooms in the house during the dead of winter, 2002.

When Valen and I were taken on a tour of the House by one of the six full-time and nine part-time staff members, we saw a beautiful,

Wearing her prized kidney necklace, Valen visits Baltimore's Ronald McDonald House in 2007 where her parents stayed while her life lay in the balance at nearby Johns Hopkins Hospital.

bald-headed child happily playing with a toy in a games room while her parents watched TV nearby. It seemed so normal. And it was. Everyone there was fighting a battle, but there was a sense of comradeship, of closeness, of shared emotions that was felt by everyone, even two wide-eyed visitors.

If Ronald McDonald House was the safe haven for Valen's mom and dad, the hospital was the battleground.

With no kidneys to filter wastes from her blood and excrete them along with water as urine, Valen began daily treatments of dialysis that began immediately after both kidneys were removed on January 25th. She was immediately dialyzed for eight days straight before starting a routine of treatments three times a week. Each session lasted four to five hours each, depending on her blood pressure and other criteria, but complications were mounting. On February 4th, Bill held a container while his daughter vomited blood into it. There was also blood in her stool, so she was whisked back into the ICU. Valen would tell me years later that it helped her to look into the strong, warm eyes of her father to gather the strength she needed to hang on.

On her nineteenth birthday, Valen underwent her first endoscopic procedure. It was a minimally invasive diagnostic procedure whereby a tube with a miniature camera attached was maneuvered down her throat and into her stomach. Unfortunately, there was too much blood in her stomach for doctors to see anything to make a medical diagnosis.

No one sang "Happy Birthday."

The next day, an attempt was made to flush or suction the blood from her stomach to study the immense clot. The attempt failed. A larger tube was utilized for the second endoscopy, but still nothing could be seen because of the vast quantity of blood in her stomach.

Unfortunately, Valen remembers this unsuccessful attempt vividly. "I woke up during this procedure," she told me years later. "I remember it distinctly. During my stay at Hopkins I had a pain button that I could press, and when I did a shot of pain medicine would be administered immediately. It was used to keep a steady amount of pain medicine in my system at all times but it also had limits so I could not overdose accidentally."

Valen said she awakened during the examination but because a tube was in her mouth and throat, she could not speak. So, she ingeniously raised her hand and pretended she had the pain button. "I kept pressing this imaginary pain button with my thumb, up and down, up and down, to indicate I was pressing a pain button and to let them know I was awake and in excruciating pain. She was experiencing anesthesia awareness. Or, unintended intra-operative awareness. The action worked. Sort of. When the anesthesiologist saw her eyes open, there was no doubt what was happening. However, Valen was told to "bear with us" because she had been given enough anesthesia for an overweight, grown male and more could not be administered without hurting or even killing her.

On the next try on February 7th, they brought out the big guns. The biggest tube ever utilized for an endoscopic procedure in the hospital was put to work. The operation attracted the attention of just about everyone who worked in the intensive care unit. They came to watch, listen, and learn. The process worked this time, and it was determined that she had a congenital anomaly. It was discovered that a bleeding vessel in her stomach was pumping blood into her stomach with every heartbeat. They also discovered several bleeding ulcers in her stomach. Two clamps were attached to her bleeding stomach. She had received eleven units of blood in the past twenty-four hours. Her body holds seven units. The internal bleeding could have been caused by the thinning of the stomach lining because she had not been eating, due to pancreatitis. But it's also possible the stomach lining had been scratched by a tube that was placed in her nostril, passed down the pharynx through the esophagus, and into her stomach.

A day later, on February 8th, just two weeks after her kidneys had been removed, doctors performed emergency surgery. They re-opened the incision; cut through the stomach wall, repaired the vessel, and re-stapled the stomach incision. That night, Bill and Pam prayed because they weren't sure they'd be seeing their daughter the next day. The Covers are Christian. They are not regular churchgoers, but they have faith and they believe in God. "We prayed that night," Bill said.

February 14, 2002 was just another day in the life of Valen Cover. She felt dizzy early that morning. She was vomiting blood and blood was in her stool. And she was angry. It had nothing to do with her distressing medical condition. Her father was always in her room first thing in the morning. Every morning! No exceptions.

Pam, usually exhausted from late nights at the hospital—sometimes staying until eleven p.m.—would often remain in bed in the morning at Ronald McDonald House, not wanting to face another day of heart-wrenching drama filled with so much pain and suffering in the eyes and frail body of her little girl. Like Bill, Pam had no choice. She always dragged her weary bones out of bed and made her way to the hospital later in the day, taking what became known as "the second shift." But Bill was always there to see Valen wake up in the morning. Sometimes he would rise early and do laundry before driving to the hospital. He always arrived at Valen's room on time every day. A shuttle bus was available for residents of RMH, but Bill had his car, so he did not have to wait for a bus. By driving himself directly to the hospital, he was always on time. But not on this particular day.

As the minutes of the early morning hours slowly ticked by, Valen became more and more agitated. "Where IS my dad?" she demanded to know of any staffer who entered the room. No one knew. This was not like Bill. The Old Testament tells us there is a time for every purpose under the heavens; a time to be born and a time to die . . . Bill's purpose was to be with Valen every morning and to be on time.

"It was like a job," he would later say. "I felt it was my mission to be there at the same time every morning. It was something she could count on. Once the staff got to know us, we were given special privileges, so I always arrived a few hours before regular visiting hours." Some days he would paint her toenails purple. Other days it would take practically the entire day to get her to brush her teeth because there were so many bouts of nausea; various medical procedures by doctors; nurses administering medication; and dozens of other things that go on in the hospital room of a very sick patient. One of Pam's regular habits was to wash Valen's hair in a small, portable basin that she had used after the back surgery. Pam had used the same container at Hershey Hospital when Valen had a port inserted to deliver nutrients, and she continued to contend with it when the dialysis port was inserted at Hopkins, and right up until she received her transplant. Pam feared Valen could develop an infection from soapy water in a shower, or just by getting the ports wet.

One morning, Bill arrived to discover that Valen was not in her room. Just as panic was beginning to set in, he was informed that she had taken a turn for the worse and had been rushed to ICU in the middle of the night. She recovered. For one more day. Until the next emergency.

But on this particular Thursday morning, the fourteenth day of the month and day sixty-six of her JH stayover—Bill was nowhere to be seen. It was well after ten a.m. when he finally arrived in the room. He had been shopping. His arms were loaded down with red Valentine's Day balloons. Valen was overjoyed to see him. She glanced at the clock and in her elation, cried out with a mixture of joy and fear: "Where were you?"

When I first heard this story, I asked Valen why she reacted the way she did. "They were all I had," she replied, surprised at the question. "I had no one else but my parents. I lived for their love and support."

Bill was visibly touched by her remark. "We never abandoned her," he said, emphatically. "Never!" He paused and added, thoughtfully: "We probably dedicated ourselves to her more than was necessary, even to the extent that it hurt me and Pam emotionally."

The day after Valentine's Day, she was readmitted to the ICU. She endured another endoscopic procedure. A shot of epinephrine (adrenaline) was given to help stop bleeding ulcers that had formed around the stomach incision. She was given three units of blood and developed an allergic reaction to one of them. A breathing tube was inserted down her throat for the procedure. Her eyes, her throat, her face, all swelled. She was placed on twenty-four-hour dialysis the following day, and on February 18th, they began feeding her sugar water through a pic line—a form of intravenous access—into her stomach.

Times like this were especially hard on her parents, and they felt guilty leaving their daughter even after being with her for a dozen hours or more. "At the end of the day, our heads were hanging," Bill said. "We were fried. We would make our way back to Ronald McDonald House and we didn't know how we could go through it all again the next day."

Pam revealed to me, almost shamefully, that Ronald McDonald House was like a shelter from the storm. Pam would not eat in front of Valen, because Valen was being fed nutrients through the pic line. "We would sometimes take the crackers off her tray, save them, and eat them on the way back to the House."

They practically salivate when they speak of the meals that were prepared for the guests at Ronald McDonald House by volunteers. "Dinner was like party time," conceded Bill. "We felt bad leaving Valen in the evening, because she was lying in a hospital bed unable to eat, and we were going to enjoy a home-cooked meal. She was in such a horrible situation, but we returned to the House and tried to enjoy dinner with other adults before going back to the hospital for the rest of the evening."

Bill and Pam became very close to some of the residents, because everyone was going through a similar form of hell. Pam speaks kindly of a woman named Nora whose daughter was in the hospital suffering from anorexia. "Nora always felt that Valen would pull through," Pam remembered. "She would go to the Catholic Church down the street from Ronald McDonald House and pray for her daughter and for Valen as well."

There was one other couple Bill and Pam became attached to. They had seen them at Hershey Hospital and now they were living under the same roof with them in Baltimore. The young and attractive husband and wife had three small children. One child was a patient in the pediatric ward of the cancer wing. The husband was a pastor in Hershey. Pam first met his wife while doing laundry at the House. "After that day, we would always ask how each other's child was doing," Pam reminisced. "Of the two children, I would have guessed at the time that Valen would be the one not to survive. One evening, Bill and I were talking to the woman in the dining room area on the second floor of the House. She told us how her son responded that day with a smile. That meant the world to her. She was so hopeful. It was so hard for her to bear his pain. The next day, we heard that her son had died. We were devastated."

Pam went to the hospital later that day, carrying the burden of the child's death in her heart. Incredibly, in that enormously large hospital, she spotted the couple as they turned around a corner and entered the parking garage with their children. Pam resumed her story for me: "I felt like I was the only one there who knew the extraordinary pain this family must be feeling. They came to this hospital with three children and they were leaving with two."

The young mother saw Pam in the distance. Their eyes locked. Pam approached and embraced her. "I felt oh so sorry for her. Why one and not the other? Why not save both? Only God knows."

6

The Struggle Continues

*"Out of suffering have emerged the strongest souls;
the most massive characters are seared with scars."*
— *Edwin H. Chapin*

By winter 2002, Valen had amassed a road map of scars that criss-crossed north, south, east, and west along more than forty inches of her slender body (as measured by her mother). Yet, the incredible epic saga of her lengthy struggle with sickness and operations had no apparent effect on her good and decent nature.

I wanted to find out what sort of patient Valen was, so I spoke to some of the people who cared for her during the sickest hours of her life. I visited the intensive care unit (ICU) of Johns Hopkins in 2007 and met with several staffers who, as it turned out, not only remembered the blonde teenager they had treated in 2002, they adored the young woman who was so critically ill for so long.

Robin Karlin has worked at JH for eleven years, seven of them in the ICU ward, and she admitted that her special compassion for Valen came from "the mother in me." Valen stops by the ICU ward occasionally, whenever she is having blood work done at JH or is there for a doctor's appointment, just to visit with her former nurses. "Valen was so cute and she is so beautiful now," said the red-haired nurse. "She touched my heart with her beautiful spirit. She had—and still has—a beauty, a spark, a spirit, and vibrancy unlike any other patient I've known. She is truly one of God's Angels. I'm so glad our paths crossed."

Robin said she has a place in her heart "for the special people" and Valen has obviously left a lasting impression on the seasoned nurse.

The hospital's ICU is a controlled but busy environment; I wanted to talk longer, but I sensed I was taking Robin and her colleague, Mandy Schwarz, from their appointed rounds. Both gave me their home phone numbers and asked me to call them later. They had more they wanted to say about their former precious patient.

When I reached Robin at her home on a Monday evening, a few days later, she said Valen was by no means perfect. "She had her moods—who wouldn't, considering what she was going through?" Robin sympathized. "But she has such a sweet and endearing spirit, on the rare occasions when she was cranky toward us, she would apologize afterwards, saying over and over again: 'Oh, I'm sorry, I'm so sorry.'"

One particular incident sticks in Robin's mind that remains as fresh today as it did on the night and early morning in question in January 2002. A breathing tube was inserted in Valen's throat and remained there for over sixteen hours. It assisted her breathing during a surgery and was left there afterwards because she was not strong enough to breathe on her own. Robin had been treating her for a very brief time and had never heard Valen speak, because of the apparatus. "I wanted to see the whole package," is the way Robin put it. "I was eager to hear her speak." On this night, Robin was working the overnight shift and she was determined to stay with Valen until the tube was removed and she could hear her voice. "I was with her in the morning when she awoke and the breathing tube came out," Robin remembered. "She looked like an angel, and when she spoke, she sounded like an angel."

Before his death in 1662, St. Francis de Sales wrote: "Make friends with the angels, who though invisible are always with you." Valen's spiritual angels may have been imperceptible to the human eye, but another angel of mercy who hovered about her constantly was Robin's co-worker, Mandy Schwarz, whose thick brunette hair falls to her shoulders. After chatting with her in a hallway of the ICU ward, outside the spacious, equipment-laden room once occupied by Valen, I called her at her home on a weekday evening. Mandy spoke compassionately about her former charge. "She was struggling and in so much pain, I just wanted to hug her all the time," said the professional caregiver, who has been nursing at JH for sixteen years. "One time she was bleeding from her stomach and she was so critical, it was scary for all of us. At that time, we were worried she was not going to make it, but even though she's tiny, she's tough, and she pulled through once again."

One of the qualities that impressed Mandy most was the "character and nature" of the young woman from York. "She cared about us! She was so gracious about the care we gave her. There was no need for her to care about us, that's what we are—caregivers and that's what we get paid to do—but she was so generous in her gratitude and so kind to us." Mandy ended the conversation with a comment she reserves for the few patients who make such an indelible impression. "I look forward to her future."

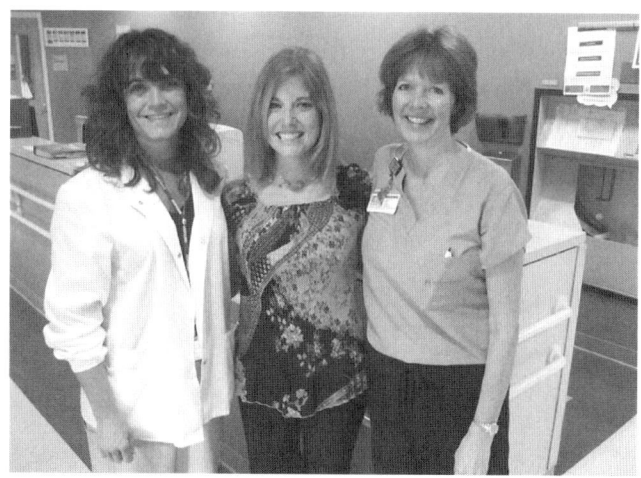

Valen's ICU nurses Mandy Schwarz (left) and Robin Karlin.

I witnessed first-hand the mutual love Valen and her nurses have for each other when I accompanied Valen on a return trip to JH one summer day in 2007 for a series of visits to hospital staff that had cared for her in the past. I knew that she had a special affinity for many of her former nurses, but there was one nurse I did not meet, and I regret it, but Valen does not even know her name. They met very briefly and it wasn't at Johns Hopkins. Valen will never forget her. She was young, blonde, and pretty. Not unlike her patient. Her job was to take a blood culture from a vein in Valen's arm. Valen noticed right away that the nurse had just one hand. She was wearing a sterile glove on her good hand and a similar glove on a "nub." Valen knew that taking a blood culture requires more dexterity than merely taking a blood sample because tubes and blood bottles have to be prepared and multiple samples need to be taken—in this case, four sets. Valen thought to herself: "This should be interesting."

At first, Valen was apprehensive, so she let it be known that most nurses have a very difficult time drawing blood from her because her veins are so small. The remark was acknowledged with politeness. Valen's interest soon turned to fascination as she watched the woman work quickly and efficiently with her one good hand. Then, out of respect, Valen turned away, not wanting to stare.

Many thoughts clouded Valen's mind. "I wonder what happened. I want to ask but I want to respect her privacy. It's so unfair. She is so young and pretty. I can hide my scars with clothes but she cannot hide her disability."

Valen prepared herself for a long session because if history were any indication, this nurse would poke and pry and stick the needle in and out and then try another area of the arm, seeking a good, blood-flowing vein. To her astonishment, the one-handed nurse stuck the needle in once, got a good vein, and before long the venipuncture procedure was over, and she was packing up the full bottles of blood samples and readying them to be taken to the lab for testing.

Valen looked at her and spoke just two words. "Quite impressive!"

"Thank you," the young professional replied, and walked toward the door. They smiled at each other. "She knew what I meant," Valen said when she related the story later. "I wanted to say so much more to her, but that's all I needed to say. She knew. Pretty cool! Pretty neat!"

Not all of Valen's favorite nurses were of the Florence Nightingale variety. Bob Cogley was one of her dialysis nurses at Hopkins who became a much-revered and necessary extension of Valen's blood system. More than two years after her successful kidney transplant, Valen visited Bob at the hospital. That visit would have a profound effect on the life of the now sixty-two-year-old nurse who made a career-altering decision when he saw her looking so radiant and healthy.

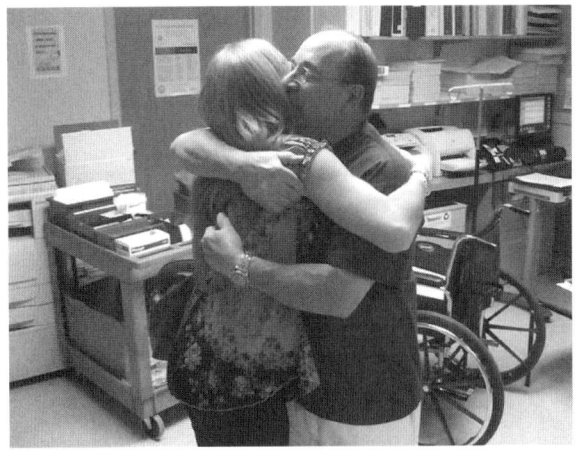

Dialysis nurse Bob Cogley gets a big hug from his former patient five years after her transplant.

He related the details to me five years after he last dialyzed her. We talked for forty-five minutes in a break room down the hall from the hospital's dialysis unit, where he works with as many as thirteen colleagues who perform an average of 800 monthly treatments. The diminutive gentleman sat at the opposite end of the lunchroom table wearing a burgundy hospital smock over loose-fitting, white cotton sweatpants. Valen and Kris sat between us. Kris was operating the microcassette tape recorder while I asked questions and took notes. In three-quarters of an hour, Bob looked at me twice. Three times tops. He was not being disrespectful. He is a kind, soft-hearted man who has been a dialysis nurse since 1973 and has been at JH for over seventeen years. He just could not take his gaze off the young woman sitting next to him who was at opposite extremes to the frightened young woman he had treated a half-decade earlier.

For two months at Hopkins, sometimes daily, but usually three times a week, for four to five hours Valen underwent hemodialysis, whereby her blood was pumped through the blood compartment of a dialyzer, exposing it to a semipermeable membrane. The cleansed blood would then be returned via the circuit back to the body. "Dialysis is the only process in medicine that changes the entire metabolism of the body in the first thirty to forty-five minutes," explained Bob.

I asked him to describe his patient of 2002. He adjusted his glasses and, while peering intently into Valen's eyes, he cast his mind's eye to the not-so-distant past. He explained that she was very inquisitive, always asking what he was doing and why. He loved that she was a "whyer" and she appreciated that Bob was not a "becauser." Valen would ask: "What does that thing do to me?" And: "Why are you holding a syringe? Are you giving me something or taking my blood?" Bob patiently explained every procedure to his young patient because he believes each patient should know what is happening to his or her body. Valen said Bob described the dialysis process to her in detail and he was truthful and frank about it. "I don't like things that are sugar-coated," she said. "He gave me the facts and was realistic about what it would be like and what I should expect. Bob was always there. He was like a father figure to me. He was a constant for me during a tough time. Constant is nice when you are sick," she smiled. Bob laughed at the recollection. "I watched her like a hawk and she watched me like a hawk."

On a particularly cold January day in 2005, Valen was at Hopkins for a checkup when she dropped by the dialysis unit to see Bob. It took her former dialysis nurse a few moments to realize who it was. When it dawned on him that it was Valen, he was startled by her healthful and wholesome appearance. She was like a ray of brilliant sunshine. He remembered her sickly, waif-like appearance the last time he had seen her. She was no longer the feeble and frail person who was sick of being sick. He regained his composure, welcomed her with a bear hug and within moments of greeting her, he made a decision that would affect his life. Valen would not hear about it until 2007.

When Bob saw his former patient on that wintry day in 2005 for the first time since she had left Johns Hopkins on March 26, 2002—the day she received her last dialysis session at Hopkins—Bob was making plans to give up his career as a dialysis nurse. He wanted to do something different with his life. In July 1971, he married Dawn, who had a hereditary kidney disease called Vitamin D-resistant rickets. She gave birth to a son in 1972, and a year later, Dawn was on dialysis. She received a life-saving kidney from her mother in 1978—an operation that was performed at Johns Hopkins. Life was good, but Dawn died in 1995 of a suspected heart attack. Bob loved his work, but he had been a lonely man for a long time. He thought a career change would give him a new lease on life. Bob made a momentous decision at the beginning of 2005. He decided to leave patient care and accept a position with a firm as a biomedical technician. "I was hired and the paperwork was completed." But that very same day, he saw Valen for the first time since her transplant and her release from JH. It had been well over two years, but when he saw her radiant smile as she entered the dialysis unit, he knew that his decision to leave this kind of work was totally wrong. "Moments after seeing her, I knew this is where I belong," he said. "When I looked at her and when I heard she was working full time, organizing fundraising walks for PKD, and going on speaking tours for PKD—and, oh, she looked so beautiful—I was in awe of what she was now doing."

I heard a clicking sound from my tape recorder, indicating that the forty-five-minute tape had come to an end. Bob kept his gaze on Valen in the cramped break room, and her eyes welled up with tears. Valen believes in the expression: "The eyes are the windows to the soul," and I could see that her eyes and Bob's were locked in unison and they revealed an attachment that only a patient and her caregiver can know. "When I first met her, she was a very sick and scared child," Bob recalled, still gazing into her large, brown, doe eyes. "She had so many bloody cysts on her kidneys. I had never encountered a patient who had undergone so much adversity at such a young age. She was looking death in the face."

Bob's epiphany on that fateful, post-transplant day was sudden and totally unexpected. "When I saw the beautiful and healthy woman standing before me after her transplant, I realized I had played a small part in her being alive. I realized then and there that I could not do anything else in my professional life, other than dialysis. So I ripped up the paperwork and here I am."

Bob's personal life has taken a positive turn. He has met a woman and has found love again. He also rides horses as often as he can in his spare time.

The poet Wordsworth wrote of "the soothing thoughts that spring out of human suffering; in the faith that looks through death." On Sunday, February 24, 2002, the only soothing thought to enter the mind of Valen Cover was that she was not scheduled to be strapped to a dialysis machine for several hours that day. She hadn't had solid food for months, so she tried eating food, but it did not go down well. "It was like swallowing a razor blade," she said, wincing at the memory of the raw feeling in her throat.

These days, Valen takes her victories and pleasures in small doses, living for today and enjoying the simplicities of life. She savors a trip to Starbucks for a Caramel Frappuccino or a fat-free pomegranate and blueberry sherbet; or she'll take delight in a drive to the Dairy Queen to indulge in a decadent Oreo Cookie Blizzard. Valen is a proponent of the Charles M. Schulz (*Peanuts*) philosophy that "Life is like an ice-cream cone; you have to lick it one day at a time." And that's the attitude to which she and her parents resigned themselves in the ongoing and long-suffering battle to regain some semblance of health. One day at a time, Sweet Jesus, as the song goes. One day at a time.

There was little to laugh about on the adult floor of the hospital where Valen spent the entire 105 days, but no one ever died of laughter, so the Covers took their humor where they could get it. One day, Valen's father asked if she would like to be wheeled outdoors. No-brainer.

Valen hadn't seen the sun or felt the exhilarating rush of cold air on her face in a month of Sundays. She was suffering cabin fever. Despite the freezing winter temperature, she was placed in a wheelchair and bundled in a warm blanket. "We could get in trouble over this," Bill warned his fresh-air-starved daughter. "I don't care," she responded, haughtily.

It was a crisp, sunny day as Bill attempted to maneuver the chair over a bumpy sidewalk without jarring his passenger or dislodging the attached IV pole. As father and daughter laughed about it years later, they realized how ridiculous it must have looked to passersby when the chair was moving forward and, at one point, the pole started to go backwards. "I was strapped to both chair and pole, and poor Dad is frantically trying to grab onto the pole as I start to roll down a hill." Humorist Will Rogers said everything is funny as long as it's happening to someone else. Bill admitted it was probably a funny scene. "It wasn't pretty, but we pulled it off," he said, adding reflectively: "We did have some journeys!"

As the snows of February made way for the ides of March, there was no indication that healthy days for Valen were on the horizon.

March 1, 2002, was a particularly bad day. Valen's blood pressure was 220/125. Her dialysis session was halted early when the machine clotted. She had been given four bags of blood, and during the last bag Valen was given 25mg of Benadryl to treat a rash that had developed on her chest, stomach, neck, and face. She had a fever and, by seven o'clock that evening, she was experiencing severe cramps. The spasms continued to plague her into the next day. On the third day, cramps in her legs and shoulders prevented her from sleeping. The battle raged on.

Dialysis continued, and in that first week of March, despite stomach pain, nausea, constipation, and the recurring rash, Valen began to eat solid food. On March 12th, she was able to eat a half bowl of Frosted Flakes, with six ounces of skim milk, and she drank four ounces of water. One small victory.

On Thursday, March 14th, she ate more cereal and drank a Nepro shake — a therapeutic, nutritional, milkshake-like drink for people on dialysis. She threw it up, but felt well enough to go for two short walks.

The list of medications Valen was now taking looked like a pharmacy's inventory. There were pills to treat high blood pressure, something for nausea and vomiting, and others for pain management. They included: Dulcolax, Clonidine patch, Epogen, Erythromycin, Fentanyl, Iron, Hydralazine, Labetalol, Reglan, Procardia, Zofran . . . and more.

The meds were just what the doctor ordered because, despite dizziness, severe cramps, and bowel problems, there was light at the end of this tunnel. On March 18th, she drank soup for lunch, and for supper she consumed a half submarine sandwich and kept it down. The next evening, she pigged out on a large portion of meatloaf and mashed potatoes. At 125.5 pounds, she would not any time soon become a spokesperson for a fast-food restaurant, but there was every indication that she would soon be well enough to return home and continue taking dialysis at York Hospital while she waited for a kidney transplant.

Her nutritional needs at the time were in the capable hands of Dennis Myers, Clinical Dietitian Specialist in the Department of Nutrition at JH Medicine. I met the slight, affable, food specialist in a hallway at JH and we talked for such a long time about Valen and her diet, he finally suggested we go to the cafeteria, have a coffee, and sit while we chatted. He lamented that Valen was among the youngest PKD patients he had ever seen with such severe kidney problems. He talked about her special dietary needs and admitted that his biggest worry was that she could contract a bacterial infection from some foods. He kept her away from unpasteurized cheese, for example, and long after he was her nutritionist, he was also advising her to drink up to five glasses of water a day, consume green tea, keep to a low sodium diet, and stay away from saturated fats. He also encouraged her to take part in moderate exercise — such as

Valen's Clinical Dietician Specialist at Johns Hopkins, Nutritionist Dennis Myers.

swimming and walking—and even gave the green light, years after her transplant, to drinking alcohol in strict moderation.

Valen went home from the hospital on Tuesday, March 26, 2002. Following one final dialysis session at Johns Hopkins, Pam wrote one word in her daily journal in large, capital letters: RELEASED. Next to that was a drawing of a "happy face." ☺

Valen was pleased to be going home, but she looked forward to a return visit in the not-too-distant future—for a lifesaving kidney transplant.

The transient college student was back home once again. She was very thankful that she wasn't sucking daisy roots, to put it indelicately, but when other nineteen-year-old females were getting prettied up and hitting the bars and nightclubs of York on Saturday evenings, Valen was heading off to 308 St. Charles Way, site of the Dialysis Center of York. And on Tuesday evenings. And Thursdays, too. Four to five hours at a time. For four and a half months.

"I didn't want to be there," Valen told me on a nostalgic, return visit many years later. "It was the hardest . . . the *hardest* thing ever! I hated the noise of the machine, but I knew it kept me alive, so I treated it like a job. A job that had to get done and over with so I could get out of there."

When I asked how she passed the time during dialysis she said she neither read nor talked to anyone. "I just practiced mind over matter and focused on the job to be done." On occasion, she would listen to music on her headphones. One time she remembers watching with envy as an elderly man ate crackers and peanut butter. Valen was vomiting her food frequently, and she loved crackers and peanut butter, but they were on her forbidden list of foods.

She remembers with fondness her dialysis nurse and consoler, Josie Seitz, who met with me and Valen on a summer evening in 2007 at the Center that was currently treating 200 patients. "She was trying at times," Josie said, as she cast a smile at Valen. "Sometimes she would cry and sometimes she would shout. But a large part of my job is to talk and to understand. I spent a lot of time talking to Valen and understanding and just keeping her company. We don't see many PKD patients as young as her, so there was an emotional impact on me and our staff, seeing one as young as her on hemodialysis and with so many other teenage issues and illnesses to deal with."

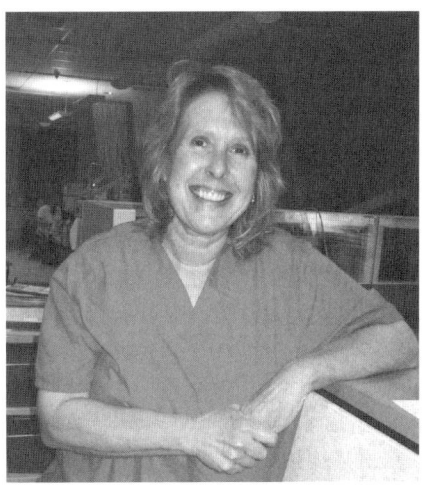

Josie Seitz was Valen's dialysis nurse at the Dialysis Center of York for over four months in the spring and summer of 2002.

Josie is no rookie. She has been a dialysis nurse for thirty-two years. She had dialyzed Pam's mother and brother. And she likes it when former patients, like Valen, return for visits. "When I see them looking so healthy, I know I've accomplished something."

Valen said she had no good memories of dialysis. "But Josie was comforting. And I was demanding," she admitted.

Other sources of comfort, besides family members, were friends like her long-time girlfriend, Ashley, and a male friend who would often rub Valen's feet while she sat in the large, green, leather armchair, the dialysis machine and dialyzer removing wastes and extra fluids from her body and then returning the cleansed blood back into her body. Valen experienced severe cramps in her feet and could not "walk them out" because she was strapped to the dialysis machine, so his foot massages were very welcome. One evening, he brought in a large bag. Something was moving inside the bag. It made a noise. "Meow." Josie knew about it and even authorized entry to the visiting kitten. The kindly gesture by Josie and the visitor made the ailing young woman grin like a Cheshire cat.

As we left the Kidney Dialysis Center, Valen was uncharacteristically quiet. She broke the silence with a startling comment. "Next time I'll do home treatment."

"Next time?"

"Transplanted kidneys don't last forever. Mine could quit working today, tomorrow or next year."

The call came when she least expected it.

On Friday, April 5, 2002, Valen was feeling nauseous, so she took Zofran. Her blood pressure was 133/93 and her pulse was 85. At six p.m. she ate a turkey burger and some jelly beans, and then vomited. She was lying on the sofa of the family living room watching TV when the phone rang. It was Sally Robertson, the mother of Valen's high school friend and college roommate, Emily.

"We are a match!" Those four little words were the loveliest Valen had heard in her entire lifetime. She was stunned. Speechless. And no words could ever express her feelings when Sally spoke again. "I want to donate my kidney to you." Her message was as pleasing as the blossoming roses of April. After her winter of discontent, Valen was being offered a gift of new life.

Much work and many tests and intricate scheduling had to be done before the transplant could take place. Meanwhile, although her pancreatitis had improved considerably, Valen was still vomiting regularly and she habitually wore the pain patch. Her blood pressure readings were very high. Eleven days after Sally's welcome phone call, Valen awoke at four a.m. and vomited. She tried to speak, but according to her mother, she was not making any sense. Pam called 911. When the ambulance arrived with Valen at the Emergency Room of York Hospital, Valen had a seizure. Her head turned to the far left, her eyes flickered, and her hands flailed in jerky movements. When it was over, it happened again. She was given a brain scan as well as a CAT scan of her abdomen.

She was taken to the third-floor care unit. Room 3460 would become her temporary home.

The seizures continued, but soon she was well enough to return home and continue with her dialysis treatments. Pam continued to monitor, administer, and record Valen's meds and meals. Her daughter's food intake on Sunday, May 5th, included two "dippy" eggs (sunny-side up), one granola bar, popcorn, meat loaf, and a baked potato. Three significant events on Thursday, May 9th, were considered momentous enough to warrant a special exclamatory sentence in Pam's daily journal for her daughter/patient: "Pooped three times!"

April passed into May and May slipped into June. As Sally and Valen awaited word on a transplant date, Valen's daily and weekly routine was becoming monotonous: Take medicine every day. Remove Clonidine pain patch from her chest every seven days and apply a new one to the skin. Check blood pressure several times a day. Take Tums with every meal. Dialysis three times a week.

But other events were occurring outside 3271 Susquehanna Trail. The world was unfolding as it should:

May 30, 2002, the final piece of debris from The World Trade Center was removed from Ground Zero. At ten p.m. and again at eleven p.m. on that date, Valen took her medication, including 40mg Protonix, 100mg Dilantin, 200mg Labetalol, and others. As a giant spotlight lit up a massive graveyard in New York City that night, Pam Cover turned on a night light and wrote an important reminder to herself in her daily journal: "Change Valen's Clonidine #3 patch on Monday."

June 29th: U.S. Vice-President Dick Cheney served as acting president for two and a half hours while President George W. Bush underwent a colonoscopy procedure. On that same Saturday, Valen's Epogen dosage was raised from 8,900 Units/mL to 12,300.

August 12th: U.S. Airlines declared bankruptcy in Arlington, Virginia. In York, Pennsylvania, Valen was on cloud nine that Monday: She had an early dialysis session. She changed her pain patch. She took her meds. At 11:15 p.m. her blood pressure was 132/76. She was all ready for a very important date.

August 13th: Valen would receive a kidney this morning from a woman who had known her since the age of thirteen. Today, Valen calls Sally Robertson "my better half." On March 30, 2007, Valen would address the Congressional Kidney Caucus (CKC) on Capitol Hill in Washington, D.C. and tell her audience: "Little did I know that this wonderful woman carried the missing piece required to make me healthy again. She is truly my guardian angel."

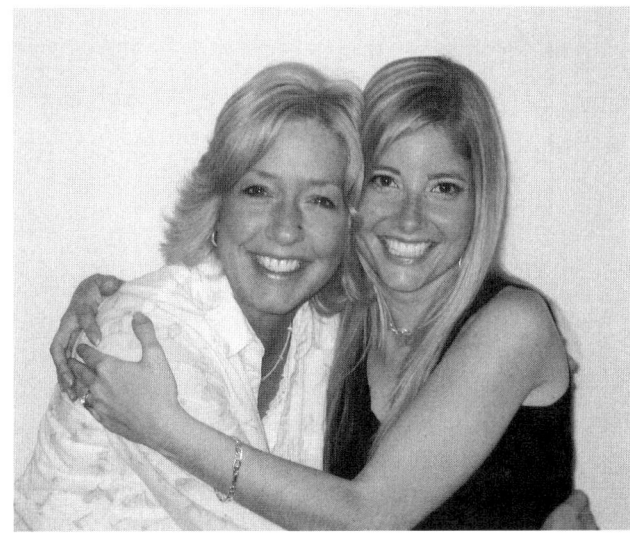

Valen and Sally at a PKD meeting in 2006.

7

The Kidney Donor

"I expect to pass through life once. If, therefore, there be any kindness I can show, or any good thing I can do for any fellow human being, let me do it now . . . as I shall not pass this way again."
—William Penn, Proprietor of Pennsylvania (1644–1718)

I knew I would like Sally Robertson, of Pennsylvania, the moment I learned that she donated her kidney to Valen. The first time I heard her name was the first time I spoke to Valen on the phone: January 18, 2006, at 8:00 a.m. During our conversation, Valen told me in her soft and melodious voice that she had received "the greatest gift of all" from the mother of a friend, in 2002. When I learned more details, I knew I had to meet this selfless person, if only for a few moments and if only to ask her one question: "Why?"

The answer to my question came on a sunny Saturday in September 2007, nearly twenty months after hearing of Sally K. Robertson (the "K" is for Knaub, her maiden name).

Four of us (Kris, myself, Valen, and Valen's boyfriend, Noah) were met at the door of the Robertsons' well-appointed home in York by a vivacious blonde wearing tartan Bermuda shorts complemented by a brown, short-sleeved top. And what a smile! It was wide as a church door. Sally embraced Valen warmly.

Valen sported a casual pair of blue jeans and a brown tunic-length top with an empire waist, gathered bodice, and scooped neckline. The lower half of her top featured bright yellow flowers, and the garment was accented by a brown, beaded, choker necklace. On her left middle finger was a heavy silver ring with eight words carved into its circumference: faith, hope, peace, happiness, inspiration, spirit, love, and trust. She and Kris had bought matching rings two days earlier at Chico's ("a clothier for sophisticated women") on York's South Queen Street. A bracelet dangled from Sally's right wrist and a silver bracelet hung from Valen's left hand. When I joked that we were part of Valen's "entourage" we were all introduced and led into the living room.

I did not have to be told that I had walked into a Christian home. Religious artifacts were in subtle evidence throughout—a cross in one room; a large, wooden sign above an entranceway that read, "*Hands to work—hearts to God*" (a previous gift from Valen); and in the dining room, a framed collage photo of the famous and inspiring ten-and-a-half-foot statue of Jesus that graces the foyer of the Johns Hopkins Billings Administrative Building.

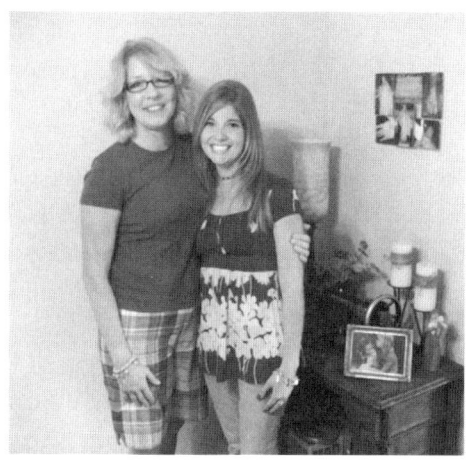

The kidney donor and recipient in Sally's house, 2007.

Before asking any deep-rooted questions, I learned that Sally was the daughter of a first assembler at the Pratt & Whitney aircraft engines plant, who helped construct the first F-16 jet engines in Florida in the 1950s. Today, Sally lives with her husband, Tim, a metal polisher, and there are five children ranging in age from eighteen to twenty-five: Emily, the oldest, Rebekah and Everett, and two stepdaughters, Ashley and Bethany.

For the past eleven years, Sally has worked at the Commerce Bank in York and is currently an administrative assistant, working for the regional vice-president of the York and Lancaster market. When she's not working, she likes to paint, but when I asked her to name her hobbies, she smiled and said her family is important to her. So is her Christianity. "I am a Christian and that sums up who and what I am," she said, adjusting the fashionable, dark-framed glasses as she warmed to a subject near and dear to her heart. "He is the reason I gave my kidney to Valen."

She had answered my question without being asked. This was why I was sitting in a stranger's house, 400 miles from my Canadian home near Toronto, Ontario. But I wanted more. I *needed* more, because I had asked myself two questions many times after knowing of Sally's altruistic act: Could I have done it? Would I do it if the opportunity arose?

"But why? You didn't even know Valen that well. She was a school friend of your daughter, Emily."

"I just knew she was a very sick young woman and if there was anything I could do to help her, I would."

Alarmed at my own temerity, I felt like the wretched Oliver Twist in the Charles Dickens classic begging for more scraps: "Please, Sally, I want more!"

She was only too happy to oblige.

"Jesus is my savior. Without him I am nothing. He has given me hope and peace beyond any understanding, and forgiveness like I don't deserve. He loves me unconditionally, in spite of myself. I wanted Valen to have a kidney and for her to know unconditional love and have her know the Lord loves her so much."

Sally looked at Valen, who was sitting across from her on a comfortable sofa, listening intently and alone in her thoughts in a room of five people.

"He never left you, Valen. We live in a broken world, in a world where bad things happen and we have terrible illnesses and diseases and people are dying and people are hurting and they may not fully understand it; but God never leaves us. He never forsakes us. He is always there and He wants us to turn to Him."

It is not the first time Valen has heard these comforting words from Sally. The two have shared their innermost thoughts since the transplant, but this day would be the first time Valen would hear some of the finer details of Sally's selfless act.

Sally was beginning to remind me of a priest I once knew at our church in Richmond Hill, Ontario. Father Henri Nouwen was a Dutch Catholic priest who wrote forty books on the spiritual life, including *The Wounded Healer* and *The Way of the Heart*. And my favorite, *Beyond the Mirror: Reflections on Life and Death,* a spiritual story of his journey of healing after a near-fatal accident when he was struck by a car while out for a walk and spent time in York Central Hospital, a few blocks from our house.

After teaching stints at the University of Notre Dame, Harvard and Yale, Fr. Nouwen moved to our community in the Toronto area and shared his life with mentally challenged people at the L'Arche community of Daybreak, about a mile from where we live. He would preach a sermon at least once a month at our church, St. Mary Immaculate, on Yonge Street, and when he did, the church was packed to the choir loft. He was such an inspired and demonstrative speaker, he would stand in the middle of the altar, literally on his tip-toes, with arms flailing to express his points. There were times I feared he would stumble and trip down the steps that lead to the main level of the church in our parish, which had celebrated its 150th anniversary in 2007. He once spoke of the love that God wants to instill in the human heart, saying: "We often confuse unconditional love with unconditional approval" and explained that God loves us without conditions but does not approve of every human behavior such as betrayal, violence, hatred, suspicion, and other expressions of evil. When he died of a heart attack in September 1996, I was surprised to see that one of his best friends was on the altar for the duration of the funeral mass. It was Fred Rogers, better known as TV's Mister Rogers, the kindly neighbor to generations of children, who died seven years later at his home in Pittsburgh, Pennsylvania.

Sally didn't stand on her tiptoes when she spoke animatedly of her decision to donate her kidney, but she did lean forward on the edge of her chair and employ her hands to express herself. "I was just the instrument for God to love Valen and give her a hope and future." She looked directly at Valen, and you could feel the love in the room. "There was never a condition for this kidney, Valen. This was a gift to you. You did not have to do or say anything to earn it, because we cannot earn God's love. It's a totally free gift." Her words reflect the teachings of German philosopher Friedrich Nietzsche, who said: "He who bestows something great receives no gratitude; for in accepting it, the recipient has already been weighed down too much."

Valen gratefully recounted how she felt when Sally called to tell her she was a match. "I was at home lying on the couch, because I was on dialysis at the time and fairly inactive. The phone rang and this sweet voice said: "We are a match!" Valen remembers feeling like the weight of the world had been lifted from her shoulders. She described it as a priceless sensation "because so many people say they want to do certain things but Sally actually had the heart to do it, and her reason is priceless and precious. After that phone call, I was happy. I wasn't scared anymore."

I asked Sally about her fear of going under the knife. I have heard that hope is brightest when it dawns from fears, but Sally was emphatic when she told me she was full of hope before the operation and had little or no fear. Most Christians believe that faith triumphs over their fears and in Sally's case it did. She didn't say it but she could easily have added that if you fear God you have nothing else to fear. That sounds like a Sallyism to me, and I'm sure she thought it. "All of my children were excited about the prospect of me donating my kidney to Valen," she revealed. "My oldest, Emily, was a little more scared than the others. My husband was okay with it if that's what I wanted to do and my parents were a little shocked. But no one ever tried to talk me out of it. No one ever expressed a negative opinion on the matter."

I was unprepared for her nonchalant response to my next question: "What did you do the night before the donor transplant operation?"

"I removed my toenail polish."

"Pardon?"

"You can't have your toenails or fingernails covered before an operation."

Valen enlightened me further when she explained that you can't have nail polish on when they put that "clip thing" on your finger to measure how much oxygen is in your blood.

Sally had noticed that Emily was a little more clingy that night. Emily joined her mother on the floor and removed her nail polish, too, in a sign of mother-daughter solidarity.

Everyone has fears, some real, some irrational. But it was revealing to hear Sally say that the only apprehension she ever felt was during the weeks leading up to the operation when she underwent a battery of tests. She was fearful that something, anything—a low blood count or a vitamin deficiency—could prevent the donation from happening. But after passing every test in the most thorough physical examination she had ever endured, she was given the green light.

On the morning of the surgery, the family left their York home at six a.m., Tim driving Sally and their daughters to Johns Hopkins Hospital, about an hour away. Sally's parents drove separately. Everett, thirteen at the time, was on a holiday with his birth father, but before he left he had presented his mother with a bouquet of roses.

When they arrived in Baltimore, Sally said she felt no anxiety. Although they were being prepped for the surgery in separate rooms, when they did see each other Valen said Sally comforted her. Sally had to go to the operating room first, to have her kidney removed. "I was a mess," conceded Valen. "What do you say to a person who is going to have an operation so you can stay alive?"

It became very quiet in the living room. You could almost hear the thump-thump-thump sound of five heartbeats. Valen choked back tears and relived the moments before the life-altering event. "I gave Sally a small gift. It was a tan-colored gemstone in the shape of a kidney. It was given to me by a nurse who had had a kidney transplant, and just before her operation, her sister gave her this gemstone as a good luck charm. I gave it to Sally because she was giving me her kidney and it was the only form of kidney that I was able to give her."

Silence is golden, and I knew at that point that my job as the interviewer was to clam up and be the proverbial fly on the wall. On the east coast of Canada, where I was born, they say: "It's so quiet you can hear the fog lift." On this sunny day in Sally Robertson's house, it was so quiet I could hear the whir of my microcassette tape recorder.

Valen continued in a composed voice. "I didn't say anything, because I was bawling. I hugged her and she whispered in my ear: 'Jesus loves you.' Then I watched her get wheeled into the operating room."

Sally broke the ensuing silence with her recollection of the moment. She remembered saying goodbye to her family and confessed it was the only time her emotions got the better of her. "I just wanted them to know I loved them. Emily was crying. Tim was a little choked up. Rebekah was okay. She was my rock."

Obviously, Sally had been in the hospital previously, to deliver her children, and once with tonsillitis, and when she'd had encephalitis as a child. She summoned up another childhood memory, when her brother was swinging her around and around "like an airplane." She had a sunflower seed in her mouth and sucked it into her lung, much like a 747 sucking a bird into its engine. Luckily the seed was extracted before lasting harm was done.

Back at Hopkins on the morning of August 13, 2002, Sally remembers feeling very cold as she was wheeled toward the operating room. The image of a long hallway is fresh in her mind today. She conjures up the memory of passing by rooms and wondering what was going on behind those doors. The brief journey ended when they placed her on the operating table. She did not see her surgeon,

Dr. Cooper, so she asked for him. When he arrived, his forty-year-old patient had something to tell him. "If something happens to me, I want you to still take out my kidney," she informed the surgeon. "If my heart fails, or whatever, please give my kidney to Valen."

The stillness in the York family living room remained. "I just wanted the doctor to know that," Sally said. "I don't know if he would have honored my request if something did happen, but I didn't want anyone else to have to worry about that."

I had one last pre-operation question for Sally.

"Did you pray?"

"Oh, yes!"

Post-operation was painful for Sally. It was more than she had expected. More painful than the birth of her son by Caesarian section. She stayed in the hospital for two days and was off work for two weeks, which is how long she said the pain lasted. She felt good, emotionally, following the procedure but when Valen's body experienced some rejection issues, Sally's mental outlook went for what she called a roller-coaster ride. She was on pain medication and remembers the feeling of immense sadness the morning after the operation when Valen called her to say she had to go back for exploratory surgery so doctors could deal with the minor rejection of the kidney. A biopsy was performed by Valen's transplant surgeon, Dr. Robert Montgomery, and she received rejection treatment. Sally vividly recalls lying on the sofa, crying. But her faith kicked in and she soon felt a sense of peace about the entire matter, knowing in her heart that God would see Valen through this ordeal.

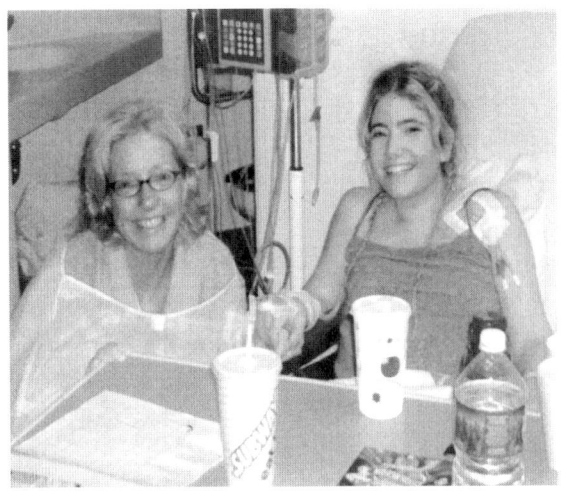

Sally and Valen after the transplant.

It was turning into an emotion-packed meeting, this bringing together of donor and receiver and three interested observers. Valen met Sally's gaze with a look that only can be communicated by two people who have shared such medical intimacy. It was as though there were just two in the room, not five. I thought of the inscription on a wedding invitation I had once seen: "And two shall become one."

Finally, Sally broke the pure silence and shared her thoughts with us. "I am sitting here looking at this beautiful young woman and thinking that I saw her at her worst. It was heartbreaking, especially when she still had her diseased kidneys. I still find it hard to comprehend. At the time, I wanted to comfort her, but what do you say? Sometimes words are of no comfort." She reached into the depths of her soul and revealed to us that we have to go through horrible trials and pain, but God brings us through trials and tribulations and when He does, our character is being formed. So is our faith and so is thankfulness.

Sally attends the non-denominational Living World Community Church on Cape Horn Road in nearby Red Lion, Pennsylvania, a community of 6,150 souls where Valen lived for awhile until the summer of 2007. The church is described as "a place to belong . . . a place to grow . . . a place to give." Fittingly, this very giving member of their congregation had asked that Valen and her family not thank her for the kidney donation. "I don't mean that in a bad way, because they have shown love and gratitude beyond measure, but I want them to know that it was my love for Valen and God's love for Valen and that's all I ever wanted for her." Sally admitted that at times it has been awkward, with some people calling her a hero. "I can understand why some people would say that, but I don't want the focus to be on me. God used me. I was the instrument. And I was willing."

I added my opinion that it was truly a selfless act. But she would not even accept that compliment. "It was an act of love and my reward was just to be a part of this blessed and awesome event. So, to me, it was not selfless."

As we prepared to leave, Sally's now-eighteen-year-old son, Everett, entered the house. I asked what he thought of his mother's decision to donate her kidney. At first he looked like a deer caught in the headlights. And who could blame him? He walked into his home on a quiet Saturday afternoon, and a book writer bombarded him with a life-and-death question. But he soon warmed to the topic and said he admired her for doing it and he knew why she did it. "My biggest fear was that something could go wrong and something bad would happen to her," he said.

Then the inevitable question: "Would you do the same, if given the opportunity?" He glanced at his mother, as if for guidance, but answered on his own. "Yes. I would like to do something like that someday."

We all smiled and nodded. Everett has a big heart. Just like his mom.

Before we left, I informed Sally that I had conducted hundreds of interviews for hundreds of stories in my long and storied career as a journalist, and there was one more question I had to ask her. "It's more of a personal request," I offered, respectfully.

She paused only slightly. "Okay."

"I have never in my career asked this of any of my interview subjects. Never! Not once!"

A nervous look appeared on her face. Her lower lip trembled only slightly. *What now?* she must have thought. She murmured, timidly, "Um . . . okay."

I eased myself out of the comfortable chair. Now I was standing next to her. She stepped back a pace. Her body language spoke volumes. "Yes? What is the question?"

"May I have a hug?"

She bestowed an appreciative smile and a generous hug that I packed away in my bag of memories. I take them out from time to time as a reminder of this special lady.

I knew I'd like Sally K. Robertson the moment I first heard about her.

8

The Transplant and the Surgeon

"It was a miraculous thing to be part of restoring you to the person you are now. You had something to do with where I went in my career, to specialize in only the most difficult cases."
— *Dr. Robert Montgomery, speaking to Valen in his office on August 31, 2007.*

Tuesday, August 13, 2002, was a happy day for the McCloskeys. Kris and I attended a family barbecue at the new home of my sister, Margie, and her husband, Brian, in Brooklin, Ontario. My brother, Wayne, his wife, Sabina, and their young son, Justin, were home from British Columbia, and my mother was there with her friend, Art, from her home north of Toronto. Nieces and nephews and other in-laws joined us for the summertime fun.

In Baltimore, a meeting of the Maryland Commission on Human Relations began at 10:05 a.m. and ended at 11:40 a.m. The city's major league baseball team, the Orioles, were in Minneapolis on August 13th losing 6–0 to the slumping Minnesota Twins in the opener of a three-game series.

U.S. President George W. Bush spent the day in Waco, Texas, hosting an Economic Forum in Jones Concert Hall at Baylor University. In a lengthy speech, he touched on several topics, including the country's medical problems. "Health care must be affordable and it must be accessible," he lectured his audience. And he spoke of the war in Iraq. "We've got a war to fight. But it's a war we're going to win." He acknowledged that the country has gone through tough times in the past, but he expressed his optimism that things would get better. "I'm incredibly optimistic about America," he asserted. "I'm confident in our spirit. I'm confident in the skill of the people."

August 13, 2002 was a typical day for most of the world's 6.6 billion people, and many went about their normal business; having barbecues, attending meetings, playing sports, and delivering speeches.

But for a young woman in York, Pennsylvania, whom I had yet to meet, it was anything but an average day. Her life would be extended on this date in history by a world-renowned surgeon, Dr. Robert A. Montgomery, and Sally Robertson, the mother of Valen's friend Emily.

Tuesday was the fourth consecutive day that temperatures reached at least ninety degrees Fahrenheit in York County, but the heat wave was the least of Valen's thoughts as she and her parents drove from their York home to Johns Hopkins Hospital where she would receive her new kidney.

Consumed with anticipation, Bill tried his best to concentrate on the road as he guided his car south along I–83 through the light, early-morning traffic during the hour-long drive to the city. Pam was quiet, lost in her thoughts of a hopeful future for Valen on this auspicious morning that was filled with so much promise. All three were optimistic, but they were also burdened with uncertainty.

Valen listened to her favorite CD and a cherished song, *Bring on the Rain*. The music of female country singer Jo Dee Messina had been an inspiration and source of comfort during months of dialysis, and on this morning in particular, the words resonated in Valen's ears:

> *Another day has almost come and gone*
> *Can't imagine what else could go wrong*
> *Sometimes I'd like to hide away somewhere and lock the door*
> *A single battle lost but not the war . . .*
> *Tomorrow's another day*
> *And I'm thirsty anyway*
> *So bring on the rain.*

When they arrived at the hospital on North Broadway, Bill steered into the parking garage. The sound of the award-winning country artist from Holliston, Massachusetts, resonated in Valen's mind:

> *It's almost like the hard times circle round*
> *A couple drops and they all start coming down*

Yeah, I might feel defeated,
I might hang my head
I might be barely breathing — but I'm not dead . . .
I'm not gonna let it get me down
I'm not gonna cry
And I'm not gonna lose any sleep tonight.

The waiting was over. Valen had been through the transplant workup process of at least ten tests, including chest x-ray, electrocardiogram, barium swallow, gastroscopy, cystoscopy, tissue typing, and various blood tests. The transplant team members — the nephrologist, anesthetist, transplant coordinator, and others — had concluded their consultations and evaluations.

The time had come.

Valen's kidney transplant surgery (also called a renal transplant) took several hours. During the operation, Sally's kidney was inserted and attached through an incision in Valen's left lower abdomen. Dr. Montgomery attached the artery and vein of the new donor kidney to the iliac artery and vein and then attached the ureter to Valen's bladder.

That's the simple, layman's version. While researching this book in 2007, I asked Dr. Montgomery for a personal, face-to-face interview to learn more about him and Valen's transplant. He said he'd love to talk to me.

Dr. Robert Avery Montgomery, MD, Ph.D., is Associate Professor of Surgery, Director of the Incompatible Kidney Transplant Program, Chief of the Division of Transplantation, and Director of the Comprehensive Transplant Center at The Johns Hopkins University and Hospital. Some say he is a medical revolutionary, and many elevate him to "star transplant surgeon" status.

He received his medical education at the University of Rochester and earned his Ph.D. at the University of Oxford, England. A member of many Surgical Societies and the recipient of important awards, distinctions, and scholarships too numerous to mention here, Dr. Montgomery is well known for his involvement in the development of innovative approaches to expanding live donor renal transplantation. He has been featured on the *Today Show, Good Morning America*, the *CBS* and *NBC Evening News, CNN*, The Discovery Channel, and in *USA Today, The New York Times, The Washington Post,* and *The Wall Street Journal.* He was part of the team that performed the world's first live donor kidney removal using minimally invasive techniques. He also led the team that performed the first triple swap kidney transplant. He is considered a world expert on kidney transplantation for highly-sensitized and ABO (blood type) incompatible patients.

The six-foot-one physician is also known for his calm, easygoing manner, trademark cowboy boots, and bushy Fu Manchu-like mustache that extends downward past his mouth and jaw line. The mustache is not unlike the horseshoe-style 'stache worn by wrestler Hulk Hogan—just longer and thicker—and it complements his light brown hair that is worn long, almost to his shoulders.

I knew of his stellar reputation long before I'd met him. On November 21, 2006, I read an article in my morning paper about a five-way kidney swap that he had choreographed on November 14th. Five kidney patients from across the country had received new organs from five unrelated living donors in what doctors at Johns Hopkins called the first five-way kidney swap in medical history. Dr. Montgomery headed the transplant team that involved six operating rooms, twelve surgeons, eleven anesthesiologists, and eighteen nurses. A total of approximately 100 medical personnel were involved in the transplants, including immunogeneticists, nursing coordinators, and pharmacists. Nine people and an altruistic donor—someone willing to give a kidney to anyone who needed it—had enough matched kidneys among them to pull off the complex, five-way swap. The donors and recipients came from Ontario, Canada; West Virginia; Florida; Maine; and Maryland. History was made again on April 5, 2008, as Dr. Montgomery led nearly 100 medical professionals at JH in the first U.S. six-way kidney swap.

The first U.S. kidney exchange occurred in 2000 at Rhode Island Hospital in Providence after two women were admitted in the same week needing transplants. Both had adult children who wanted to donate kidneys, but weren't medical matches. One mother had blood type A, while her son had type B; the other mother and her daughter were the opposite, making a paired exchange possible.

Today, Dr. Montgomery is a leading advocate of "paired kidney donations" in which pairs of incompatible donors and recipients are matched with others. Kidneys are swapped so that each donor gives a kidney to a stranger. So far, the practice is limited—more than

300 exchanges have been performed—but with 75,000 patients in the U.S. awaiting kidney transplants, kidney swapping could move more people off the waiting list.

At 11:00 a.m. on August 31, 2007, Dr. Montgomery's administrative assistant, Cinda ("Cindy") Grisbach, welcomed us to the doctor's tastefully decorated office in the Ross Building on Rutland Avenue. Joining me in Room 765 were Valen and my wife, Kris, who would operate the tape recorder.

For this occasion, Valen wore black slacks and her favorite multi-colored—turquoise, black, yellow, and rose—crimpled blouse. The top, with a flowered motif, has a high, round neckline and the stitching on the shirt's trim has the same wavy design. Around her neck she wore the kidney-shaped gem that she had given to Sally just before the transplant and which Sally had mounted on a necklace and re-gifted to Valen six months later.

We sat at a table in the center of the doctor's office and I soon learned that Dr. Montgomery had performed over 1,000 kidney transplants since 1997, but when I asked if they ever become routine, he enlightened my blind and naked

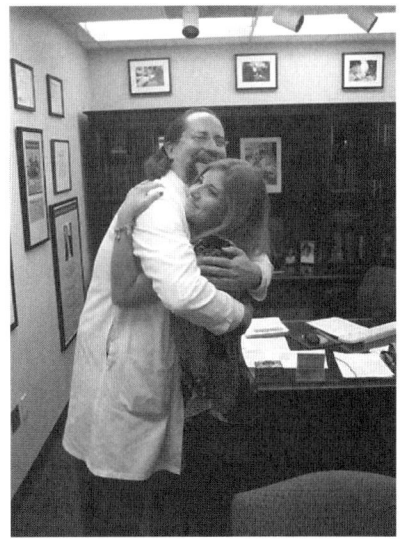

Dr. Montgomery and his former patient share a hug in his office, August 2007.

ignorance. "Not at all, Dennis! Everyone looks different on the outside just as everyone looks different on the inside. There are different challenges with each operation."

Next question: "How did Valen get so lucky to be operated on by you?"

He glanced at his former patient, smiled, and said: "I'm a sucker for hopeless cases." He said it in such a serene, sympathetic tone of voice, I knew he was not joking. He winked at Valen and addressed her: "You had been in the hospital for months, often in the intensive care unit; you had pancreatitis; terrible cyst bleeds; you had already received over seventy blood transfusions and were beginning to form antibodies; you were on dialysis; and your blood pressure was very high. Your nephrologist, Dr. Terry Watnick, contacted me. She believed you were not going to get better without a kidney transplant, but you were too sick for a kidney transplant; and, besides, there was no donor waiting in the wings. Tell me that's not hopeless!"

Dr. Watnick sought the help of Dr. Montgomery because she felt if a transplant were a remote possibility, there would be a real problem trying to find a match, so Valen might need an incompatible transplant. The Johns Hopkins Division of Transplantation performs approximately 240 kidney transplants a year, and more than ever, the Division is committed to increasing living donation through incompatible transplantation and paired donation. Dr. Watnick had come to the right doctor and the right humanitarian.

During our meeting, Montgomery's compassion was clearly visible even as he spoke of Valen's parents. "They were very young and they were at the end of the line," he remembered, as he gazed fondly at the young woman sitting next to him at the round table in his office. "They were such engaging people, they drew me in. They were so desperate and they truly thought they were going to lose you. They felt they had tried everything; you were slipping away, and this was their last resort."

He met Bill and Pam before he met Valen. And what a shock it was when the doctor met his patient for the first time!

He described Valen as someone who was depersonalized by her illness. His eyes did not stray from her as he spoke, and the three of us listened intently. "You had lost most of your hair, and you had a moon face as a result of a lot of excess fluid," he explained. "You were featureless, and I know why: you were just so tired of people hurting you, poking and prodding you, and sticking needles in you. Whenever someone came near, you reacted and regressed. You were one of the youngest PKD patients I had ever seen and you were as sick as anyone I had ever seen with kidney trouble."

He held her in his view as if looking for a sign that he should change the subject. But Valen was fascinated to hear this for the first time from her surgeon. So he carried on. "You did not respond or engage, but there was something from within you, something shining that is still present as I look at you now; some light that I picked up on. The light was there, but everything else had been stripped away by the illness. I am a very involved surgeon, but I was drawn into that drama and I got very much more involved in your case. In the end, we transplanted you in a condition that I normally wouldn't."

His next revelation came as a bombshell to all of us, but especially to Valen.

"At that time, and ever since then, I have been taking care of sicker and sicker patients, but you were fairly early on in that whole process of my career of being drawn to patients like you. It was a miraculous thing to be part of restoring you to the person you are now. You had something to do with where I went in my career, to specialize in only the most difficult cases. It was such an amazing thing. You are not even recognizable as the person you were then. You were close to rock bottom. Transplantation is a life-changing event for anyone, I understand that, but you were one of the first people for whom the drama unfolded for me like no other patient."

Valen's eyes reddened, her lips quivered slightly and she sobbed, quietly. Kris comforted her by placing a hand on her left arm. Then Dr. Montgomery reached out and held Valen's right hand, with his left. Kris withdrew but the doctor continued to gently squeeze Valen's delicate hand. No words were spoken. Immediately, Valen stopped trembling and a sense of calm overcame her. There was such a profound and obvious change in her demeanor, I asked her about it later over lunch at The Cheesecake Factory at Baltimore's famous Inner Harbor. "Dr. Montgomery has a presence that totally engulfs me," she said. "His touch and aura is smooth and gentle. I am spellbound by his intelligence, his passion for his work, and the risks that have led him to his prestigious ranking in the world."

She was about to continue when she stopped, looked down, and blushed slightly. I asked her to resume and not to be embarrassed by her extraordinary admiration for the man. She demurred for an instant before continuing. "He has this supernatural presence that surrounds him. He seems to glide and slightly float rather than walk on the ground." She looked at me and Kris to gauge our reaction. She must have felt comfortable with our empathetic feelings because she continued talking. "His confidence is striking," she added, unselfconsciously. "I am fueled by his motivation and desire to work hard and make a difference. When I am in the same room with him, I just want to be a better person."

Back in the doctor's inner office, my thoughts were interrupted by the sound of an unusual ringtone. It was the doctor's cell phone, playing a piano riff to the tune of *Bad to the Bone*, a blues-influenced rock song by George Thorogood that includes the following lyrics.

The head nurse spoke up
And she said "leave this one alone"
She could tell right away
That I was bad to the bone

The interruption allowed me an opportunity to glance around the elongated office. I spotted a book titled *The Life of Sir William Osler*, a Canadian-born physician who is often called the Father of Modern Medicine. In 1893, he was one of the first professors of medicine at Johns Hopkins School of Medicine. Two side walls of the office are covered with plaques, awards, certificates, and framed photos and letters of thanks, including one from the publicist of a world-famous race-car family who was a patient of the doctor's and whose husband is a major player in the Champ Car World Series. "They got me interested in car racing," the doctor explained, when I asked about this particular plaque on his wall. "Every year they invite me to one of the Grand Prix races and I usually go with my son, John. Last year we went to the race in Toronto."

There is other evidence of his extra-curricular hobbies and activities. On one wall is a framed front cover of *Baltimore Magazine* featuring a photo of the doctor with one of his prized alpacas. A hunter who loves the outdoors, he owns an alpaca farm where he raises the long-necked, thick-fleeced, South American camelids that are prized for the fibers of their wooly coats. He runs the farm with his ex-wife. He also has a place at Fells Point, a neighborhood in Baltimore that's located on the harbor and famous for its maritime past. He refers to this residence as a "crazy warehouse place" that he has renovated extensively.

At the far end of the room, a desk sits in front of a credenza made of cherry wood on which rests a built-in bookcase with glass doors. A photo of his athletic, lacrosse-playing teenage son, John, and seventeen-year-old daughter, Elizabeth, a dancer, sits prominently on the writing counter behind the desk and swivel chair. To the left, behind glass, is a photo of a striking and elegant black woman looking out from the cover of a book. It is Denyce Graves, recognized worldwide as an operatic superstar whose expressive and rich vocals have reverberated in the world's great concert halls and opera houses. Among her myriad credentials, Denyce sang the opening night performance of the Metropolitan Opera's 1997–98 Season as *Carmen* opposite Placido Domingo. My Chicago friend, Lois Pitalis—an inveterate fan of international theatre—has seen several productions of *Carmen* and rates Ms. Graves as the most realistic Carmen of all. "She is seductive and petulant and coy—all in one package," she gushed, several weeks after my visit to the doctor's office. Lois raved about the singer's "elegant and exciting stage presence," calling her "sensational."

When his phone call ended, the doctor apologized, saying it was his daughter who had called. I boldly referred to the photo and asked if he were an opera fan. He smiled, turned to look at the image of the woman who has played the title role in the operatic classic *Samson et Dalila,* and informed the trio of visitors that the two of them are dating. "We met on an airplane," he offered in explanation of his high-flying romance with the famous opera star. Still smiling, he added a note of self-deprecating humor: "What I knew about opera before I met Denyce, I learned from Bugs Bunny cartoons." In truth, he enjoys all kinds of music. The previous summer, he and his two children had attended the annual Bonnaroo Music and Arts Festival in Tennessee, a week-end-long concert featuring a huge variety of live music, art, and good times. "We camped out and had a great time."

I continued the interview by asking what made Valen's case so complex and complicated. He explained that it was a difficult operation—notwithstanding all of her other medical problems—because she had a lot of scarring from the kidney removal. Her kidneys were so large and they had extended all the way down to her pelvis. Also, her blood vessels were very small.

Valen remembers the day of her transplant like it was yesterday. When she awoke from her late-morning surgery, she sat up in bed and announced to everyone present that she felt wonderful. "For the first time in a long time, I felt truly alive," she said later. She was so excited that her kidney was working. "I started to pee right away," she recalled. "After a seven-month hiatus, peeing was absolutely fantastic! I kept shouting with glee: 'Mom! I can pee!'"

It was the beginning of a new life for her. Her father said the gift of a new kidney changed Valen's life, totally, giving her existence a whole new meaning. "It also gave us back our lives," he emphasized. "Dr. Montgomery and Sally didn't rescue just one person, they saved two, and maybe more."

Unfortunately, complications soon set in.

A day later, Valen was in agonizing pain. She was returned to the operating room and re-explored by Dr. Montgomery. He performed a biopsy of her kidney and although it was functioning well, there was a rejection. "Your body was telling me there was something wrong but it was not what I thought it would be," he explained to her in our office meeting. "I thought it was a mechanical problem and there might be something wrong with the kidney, but it was not that at all." Through a fortunate chance discovery—something the doctor called "serendipity"—the rejection was treated and the problem resolved satisfactorily. She was given a heavy dose of steroids; the catheter was removed; and she literally said "good riddance" to dialysis.

Valen was again feeling like a completely different person. Another new day had dawned for her. When she looked at the future, it was so bright it made her eyes burn, as her heroine, Oprah, once said.

Dr. Montgomery was not surprised by his patient's euphoria. He explained that renal failure consumes people very slowly and they don't even realize how bad they feel until they feel good again. As the toxins leave the body, the patient cannot quite believe the incredibly good feeling. Valen was ready to leave the hospital and take on the world!

In the weeks following the surgery, she was seen by Dr. Montgomery a few times for routine follow-up visits, but when he saw her more than two years after her transplant, he did not recognize her. "I almost fell over," he remarked. "I was in the hallway in the Outpatient Department and I did not recognize you. You looked great. You had to tell me who you were and I remember saying, 'Oh, my God! I don't believe it!'"

I wrapped up my hour-long interview with the doctor of a thousand transplants with a final question: "How do you measure your success as a transplant surgeon?"

His reply spoke volumes. He simply pointed to Valen. Mere words would have been superfluous.

As we prepared to leave his office that day, Dr. Montgomery asked if Valen and I would be interested in watching him perform a kidney transplant sometime. "I do two live donor transplants every Tuesday," he noted, nonchalantly. "We could schedule something like that if you are interested."

Hello-o-o?

When?

Where?

We're there!

9

The Ringside Seat

"Savin' lives! Savin' lives!"
—*Dr. Joseph Keith Melancon's*
cheerful chant while removing a kidney
during a live donor operation, October 2, 2007,
Johns Hopkins Hospital.

Valen promised she would pick me up at 5:45 a.m. for the trip to Baltimore. I waited for her in the early morning darkness on a wicker chair on the old fashioned wraparound porch of the Emig Mansion, a restored nineteenth-century manor house in the quaint village of Emigsville, near York, Pennsylvania. To call it a B & B is accurate, but seems a disservice. The five-guestroom home, built in 1810, is decorated in fine art and authentic period furnishings and is adorned with exquisite leaded and stained-glass windows, intricate moldings, elegant marble, and original parquet floors.

I was thinking of the guest who so eloquently told owners Shary Smith and Wade Lady that their unique inn is "a safe haven in a world of impersonal cold harbors," when the headlights of a car sliced through the darkness. A quarter to six. Right on time.

Valen and I were on our way to view a kidney transplant operation. As we took the ramp to Interstate 83, I presented her with Jo Dee Messina's new studio album, *Delicious Surprise*. She thanked me for the gift in her customary exuberant manner and popped the disk into her portable car CD player. The vanity license plates on the car in front of us caught our attention: HEDIDIT. We wondered who did what. We also wondered what people thought when they spotted the words on the rear license plate holder of Valen's Honda Acura: *Transplantation Works. Kidney Recipient.*

We moved at a fairly brisk pace in what was fast becoming the morning rush-hour traffic, listening to Jo Dee sing "It Gets Better." We stopped talking to hear the lyrics of track #8, "Life is Good":

I've got my two feet on the ground
Breathin' in and breathin' out
Oh yeah
Life is good
I'm gonna grab on to today
Live every minute in the way I know I should
Life is good.

I asked Valen if watching today's transplant operation would be some form of closure for her, five years after her own transplant. She set me straight in a hurry: "Closure? Absolutely not!"

Okay, I was just asking!

She reflected on my question for a bit and implied that she didn't need closure "in regards to that." She became thoughtful and initiated a serious monologue. "I don't like to pass up a challenge or a once-in-a-lifetime opportunity, which I believe this will be," she began. "It will be a challenge for me to see what my body went through and to watch the surgeon who saved my life save someone else's today."

She kept her eyes on the HEDIDIT vehicle in front of us while she spoke. "I also believe it will give me a better understanding and appreciation for what my donor, Sally, went through."

We were both unsure if we would become squeamish watching a kidney transplant operation up close and personal. I made it clear to her that my strategy would be to take a clinical approach to the procedure; detach myself from any personal feelings and merely report on what I was observing and later write about it. She conceded that the entire undertaking would be more intimate for her, but she, too, wanted to turn it into an educational experience. "I plan on taking this first-hand experience, and the knowledge I gain from it, to better explain to others what takes place during an operation of this kind." She added that she was thrilled and felt very much honored to be permitted to take part in what she expected would be "an amazing experience and one that not many people get a chance to see. When it's over, I'm sure I will chalk it up as one of my most memorable days."

As we entered the city that was coming to life on this workday Tuesday, Valen maneuvered her Acura through the streets of downtown Baltimore as she made her way towards our final destination at 720 Rutland Avenue. She drove into the Caroline Street outpatient center parking lot and found a vacant spot on Level 2. We took an elevator to the ground floor, entered a building, and walked along a long hallway before asking a security guard for directions. He very kindly led us out of the building and across the street to the Ross Building. He spoke to a colleague in a guardhouse who allowed us to pass through an entranceway. Our guide pointed us to the appropriate door and, as he saw us off, pulled out a pack of cigarettes and lit up a smoke. Perhaps it was a reward to himself for being a Good Samaritan on this day at Johns Hopkins.

We were in plenty of time for the morning's major surgical procedure. Dr. Montgomery was making his regular rounds, checking on his patients, including a man who had undergone five transplants. Members of his staff outfitted us in baby blue hospital scrubs, and we were led down a series of hallways toward the operating rooms.

Before we entered, we were given booties to fit over our shoes, a hair net, and a surgical face mask.

We were prepped and ready to go.

When we entered the small room, I counted six people, not including the anesthetized woman who was lying on the operating table, covered in a blue hospital sheet and ready to donate one of her healthy kidneys.

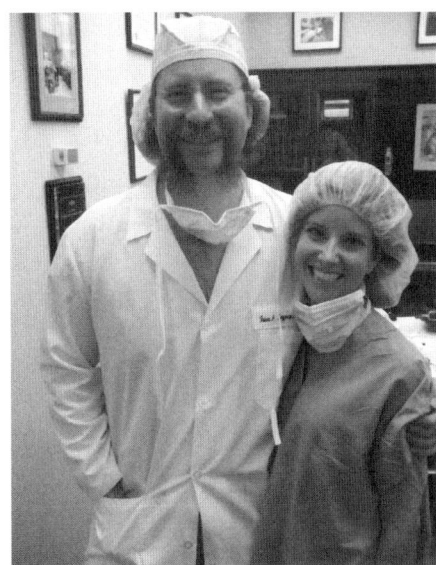

Valen scrubs up to watch Dr. Montgomery perform a kidney transplant on a female patient in October 2007.

The laparoscopic surgery had started at 8:45 a.m., before we arrived. We were introduced to the primary surgeon, Dr. Joseph Keith Melancon, aka "Big Daddy" to his friends and colleagues. The Director of Kidney and Pancreas Transplantation, and Director, Clinical Transplantation Research at the hospital, Dr. Melancon turned momentarily to greet us and then immediately resumed the task at hand. A laparoscope—a television rod lens system connected to a video camera—had been inserted in the patient's abdomen. Also attached was a fiber-optic cable system connected to a light source to illuminate the operative field.

The doctor, who was one of the participating surgeons who had made medical history by performing the first quintuple kidney transplant and was also involved in the April 5th six-way kidney swap, maneuvered the medical device as he viewed one of two large SV2 television monitors on the opposite side of the operating table. The high-definition monitors were positioned slightly above the lead surgeon's eye level and that of the assisting nurses. A third monitor faced an anesthesiologist at the head of the patient. The patient's abdomen had been insufflated—blown up like a balloon—with carbon dioxide gas to create a working and viewing space.

Almost immediately, Dr. Melancon, a Louisiana native, provided a play-by-play description of the action. "I'm following the left ovarian vein where it joins the left renal vein. The left renal vein is right about there . . . can you see it?" he asked, as Valen and I gawked first at the TV screen and then at his dexterous, gloved hands. A constant beeping sound came from one of several monitoring machines around the room. It was a good, reassuring noise, I assumed—the regular "beep, beep, beep" sound.

I glanced at Valen, who was now seated on a high stool. She looked rather pale and drawn. I stood next to her and could sense she was feeling uncomfortable. She was now looking away from the operating table. She reached for my hand and held it momentarily, for reassurance. I told her to concentrate on her breathing. "Breathe ten times. Deeply," I counseled.

I heard the doctor speak, so I approached and stood directly behind him with my microcassette recorder on high volume. "I'm just getting to the top of the kidney now." I glanced at my watch: 9:55 a.m. I stared, transfixed by what I was witnessing, as he gently nudged a firm, oval-shaped organ about five inches in length. "I'm moving the spleen away from the kidney. There's the ureter. Can you see it?" I could see it clearly on the color monitor as I simultaneously watched his hands move the devices, like he was seeking water with a divining rod. Then I spotted something, probably an artery, wiggling like a worm. "Did you see that?" asked the veteran medical practitioner. "That's called vermiculation. That's Latin for 'small worm.'" I turned to look at Valen. Her face appeared to be drained of color. I wondered if she would faint and miss the show entirely. But I was in for a surprise!

At 10:34 a.m. Dr. Montgomery entered the operating room through a door on the opposite side from where we were standing. He spotted us and shouted cheerfully: "Hi, guys. You enjoying this?"

Valen brightened immediately. It was as though her savior had arrived. He was. And he had. He had been in another operating room prepping the recipient patient and dropped by to see how the donor operation was going. After conferring with the primary surgeon and exchanging a few jokes with the nurses, he started to leave the room, turned, and addressed the transplant team: "Take your time."

Valen was now off the stool and standing behind Dr. Melancon. The color had returned to her face. The transformation was miraculous. She and I chatted quietly about the emotional event we were witnessing. We whispered, as though we were in church, but our reverence was countered by the light-hearted chatter of the medical team around us. Dr. Melancon said he'd soon be ready for Dr. Montgomery's assistance and he asked a nurse to page the surgeon. When she replied a minute later that he was not responding to the page, "Big Daddy" offered this advice: "If you want him to come immediately, send out a page with this announcement: 'Will the owner of a Shelby Cobra please come to the operating room. Your car has been hit.'"

As he worked meticulously and expertly, Dr. Melancon asked if anyone knew of a specific song by Gwen Stefani, the American singer, songwriter, actress, and fashion designer. When no one could answer his question, including me or Valen, the skilled surgeon feigned disappointment in his team. "You guys are less hip than I am!"

As he began the process of releasing the woman's kidney from the lateral wall attachment, Dr. Montgomery re-entered the room and once again conferred with his colleague on the condition of their two respective patients. "We're awaiting the results of an ultrasound," Montgomery advised Melancon.

At 11:50 a.m., Dr. Montgomery began putting ice in a small blue container in which the kidney would be placed. We could see that Dr. Melancon was cutting into flesh and we could smell burning tissue. We then observed a small amount of smoke as our eyeballs remained fixated on the screens and we watched his every delicate maneuver. A tiny amount of urine squirted from the patient's bladder. There was no tension in the room. No anxiety on anyone's part. Just a group of professionals doing their job on a Tuesday morning. Dr. Melancon broke the stillness of the moment when he sang out: "Savin' lives! Savin' lives!"

In a minimally invasive procedure, he cut an incision across the woman's abdomen about eight inches wide and six inches below her navel. He retrieved her kidney and handed it to Dr. Montgomery, who placed it in the plastic ice-filled container on a covered stand that was laden with silver-plated medical implements at the foot of the operating table.

Melancon returned to his spot and began the laborious task of closing the patient. Moments later, he stopped, turned, and walked toward Valen. "The string on my face mask is bothering me. Can you please fix it?" he asked, turning sideways. Valen grasped the string that had slid over his ear and she placed it on his head where it belonged, away from his ear. He thanked her and returned to his patient. Valen beamed like a bright beacon.

Dr. Montgomery's latex-gloved hands were immersed in the ice water as he adroitly cut and flushed the blood vessels to the kidney with a preservative solution causing the liquid in the oblong bowl to become a crimson red.

The two surgeons worked in tandem, with Melancon performing the job of closing the patient, and Montgomery preparing the donor kidney for transplant. When he was ready, Dr. Montgomery picked up the blue container and without ceremony or fanfare, headed for the exit. He called out to me and Valen. "Hey, guys. Want to come with me?"

He was the Pied Piper as we filed out of the room and walked with him and three others down a long hallway to another operating room. At the far end of the narrow hall, a nurse stood at an open door and called out in a singing voice: "Kidney parade coming!"

I walked a few paces behind Dr. Montgomery, whose careful pace was matched by Valen as she strode by his side. "I'm surprised the next operating room is so far away," she remarked. "Were Sally and I this far apart?"

The doctor, ever mindful of the treasure he was carrying, looked down at his strolling partner, smiled and joked: "No, you were nearby. I think I drop-kicked the kidney into the next operating room."

We all laughed as we entered Carnegie Room 724, aka Operating Room #4.

The melodious sound of Tom Petty's *Wildflowers* album resonated from a portable CD player. I stared at the comatose figure of a woman lying on her back on a long operating table under the glare of two giant-size Skytron skylights, with the light of five bright bulbs trained on her. A large woman, she was covered in a blue sheet similar to that of her donor, but a massive, gaping hole exposed her abdominal cavity. Five large-scale surgical clamps held back the flesh and tissue, revealing the immense chasm in the midsection of her body.

The music of Tom Petty's hit song "Wake up Time" filled the room.

> *And it's wake up time*
> *Time to open your eyes*
> *And rise and shine . . .*
> *Yeah, you'll be all right,*
> *It's just gonna take time.*

Of the eight people in the white, tiled room, only one person would not hear Petty's wake-up call. And that was a good thing. For the next few hours, Dr. Montgomery, assisted by Dr. Andrew "Andy" Singer, a second-year Transplant Fellow who also took part in the April 5th six-way simultaneous transplants, would be busy installing a kidney inside the yawning abyss.

At 12:32 p.m., Dr. Montgomery invited me and Valen to look inside the deep pit, causing Valen to recoil a bit. Her former transplant surgeon asked if this is how she imagined it. "No, not at all," said a wide-eyed Valen. "Was mine that deep?" He shook his head and explained that her kidney was inserted closer to the skin because she is such a small person.

He arranged for Valen to stand on a stool at the head of the patient so she could get a bird's eye view of the proceedings. I stood a few feet from the invalid woman's side with my tape recorder whirring silently, ready to pick up any bit of conversation from the doctors, nurses, and other attendants.

The kidney remained in the ice-filled container as Dr. Montgomery continued his preparation of the organ and the body for transplant. Like a virtuoso, he deftly clamped blood vessels so blood would not shoot out and splatter the surgeons and observers. And he prepared arteries. When he was ready, he gently lifted the chalk-white kidney—now drained of blood—from the plastic holding tray. It was wrapped in a gauze cloth and he carried it like a tiny dolphin in a sling. The woman's sleeping body rose and fell ever so slightly with each breath as the vital organ was placed inside the dorsal region of her abdominal cavity.

Coincidentally, the rocking sound of Bruce Springsteen's "Secret Garden," from his 1995 *Greatest Hits* album was now booming from Dr. Montgomery's sound machine.

> *She'll let you deep inside,*
> *But there's a secret garden she hides . . .*

Wow! Talk about choreographic timing!

Next in the surgeon's repertoire of selected and apropos tunes, was Springsteen's "This Hard Land," where he sings about staying hungry and staying alive, if you can. *"And meet me in a dream of this hard land."*

Dr. Montgomery, using a hole-punch instrument, began making holes in the arteries where he would soon connect the woman's arteries with those of the donor kidney. Wearing a microscopic light resting on the bridge of his nose, he worked proficiently with his colleague on the opposite side of the table. As their fingers worked diligently inside the woman's body, they exchanged light-hearted and good-natured teasing. Dr. Montgomery squirted a solution on Dr. Andy's hands as the latter surgeon worked swiftly with the suture in the deep hole. Montgomery was washing away blood from his colleague's hands, joking that Dr. Andy works so fast he creates friction. His partner chuckled and made a comment about spontaneous combustion.

Valen was alert and wide-eyed like never before. Her expression revealed an inquisitiveness and curiosity that, to me, was astounding. She peered so far over the blue sheet covering the head of the patient that I feared she would topple into the opening of the woman's midsection. Dr. Montgomery asked Valen if she could see okay and she assured him she could.

A nurse asked about Valen's transplant and Dr. Montgomery commented on how great she's doing. Valen spoke of some of the "fun stuff" going on in her life, all the while standing on her tiptoes so as not to miss a stitch or a single movement by the two surgeons. Her hands rested on her hips; her eyes practically popped out of their sockets. She kept edging forward on her viewing stool, her head moved left and right and her eyes darted in every direction as if keeping time with the musicality of the surgeon's swiftly moving fingers. Valen was absolutely and completely mesmerized by what she was seeing. Neither of us had taken a water break or a pee break since we entered the donor operating room earlier that morning. We did not want to miss a thing!

A nurse mentioned that she was planning a trip to Las Vegas and wanted to see "O," the *Cirque du Soleil* show at the Bellagio Hotel. I advised her to buy the cheapest seats in the house—the ninety-nine-dollar ones at the top of the cavernous room—to get the best view. Another nurse threw out an amusing, hypothetical question: "If Dennis's book is made into a movie, who will play Dr. Montgomery?"

Someone suggested Tom Selleck "in his Magnum, P.I. days when he sported a thick mustache." Dr. Andy implied that the American actor Matthew McConaughey would be perfect. Then he changed his mind and named Brooklyn-born actor Zero Mostel before joking: "Naw, forget it, he's dead."

Suddenly, Dr. Montgomery exclaimed. "Dennis! Valen! Look at this!"

He had connected the whitish donor kidney to the woman's arteries, and in seconds the lifeless organ came to life as it filled with blood and was transformed into a healthy, beet-red, living organism. Blood squirted up like a small fountain. A small amount splattered on the hospital garments of both doctors. A concerned Dr. Montgomery looked up at Valen. "Are you okay?" Once again, she assured him she was fine.

I felt I was witnessing a miracle. And I was. The miracle of transplantation. I had seen a star surgeon—a veteran of over a thousand transplants—once again turn hope into the living reality of an extended life for this seemingly lifeless woman reclining on a stark, hard, hospital gurney. Soon she would be enjoying her family and friends and no longer relying on a dialysis machine to sustain her life. Her doctor was indeed a champion of hope.

Now he had to do the "plumbing part" as he prepared to attach the kidney to the bladder. He glanced up at Valen, pointed to a machine and asked her to turn off the saline drip. She did. And once again she beamed like a thousand-watt light bulb.

At 1:43 p.m., the two doctors switched places and continued suturing. "The next hour will be boring," Dr. M. offered apologetically. Valen and I exchanged glances and smiled. We were heading into hour five of the most stimulating and enthralling day of our lives. By now, Dr. Montgomery could have read the Baltimore phone book to us and we would have listened intently and with fascination.

The workday was reaching its conclusion on a highly positive note by everyone—doctors, nurses, anesthesiologists, the writer, the former transplant patient, and especially the kidney donor and recipient whose lives were altered on this Tuesday in early autumn.

The surgeons closed the patient by stapling the fleshy abdomen. The operation ended at 2:19 p.m. Dr. Montgomery pulled the surgical mask from his face, made a call on his cell phone and chatted briefly with us before he left to tell the woman's husband that the operation was a success.

I had a question for him. "Was this just another day at the office?"

"Not at all! Every one is different."

He had a question for us.

"What are you two doing on October 21st?"

I looked at Valen. She looked at me. We both shrugged. "Nothing."

"I'm having a cocktail party at my place. Would you like to come with your partners?"

Hello-o-o?

What time?

Where?

We're there!

10

The Cocktail Party and the Society Ball

"When I first met Valen, she was a very, very sick girl. I did not think she would survive."
— Dr. Robert Montgomery, addressing ninety guests
at a cocktail party, October 21, 2007.

Interstate 83 from York to Baltimore was fast becoming a well-traveled route for Valen's Toronto-based friend/mentor/supporter/pretend dad/biographer. As we listened to her favorite CD on the way home from viewing the transplant on October 2, my musical thoughts turned to a popular folk singer, Canada's own Tom Cochrane and his signature hit song, "Life is a Highway," from his 1991 album *Mad Mad World*.

I was thinking of the life-affirming experience Valen and I had witnessed that day and I contemplated the first two lines of Cochrane's song: *"Life's like a road that you travel on / When there's one day here and the next day gone."*

The chorus reminded me of the beautiful and the brave and the strong and the young and the confident woman sitting next to me in the driver's seat:

> *There's no load I can't hold*
> *Road so rough this I know*
> *I'll be there when the light comes in*
> *Tell 'em we're survivors.*

I knew her thoughts also were on the day's extraordinary events, but she drove in silence. Then, like a bolt out of the heavens, we saw it at the same time. We were in the northbound passing lane, moving slowly in the evening rush hour traffic. We looked at each other, wide-eyed, mouths agape. It couldn't be! This was too amazing!

There are 2.6 million residents in the Baltimore Metropolitan Area. How many vehicles travel north on I-83 on a Tuesday evening just before dusk? Thousands? Tens of thousands? Incredibly, the vehicle in front of us was the very same car we followed into the city some twelve hours earlier. We shouted out the license plate aloud and in unison: "HEDIDIT!"

Neither of us believes in coincidence. Things happen for a reason. This was some sort of sign. But what did it mean? We discussed it as the traffic moved forward at a steady forty-five mph. We could think of only one explanation. Crazy as it sounds, we agreed that it had something to do with the events of the day at Johns Hopkins. We had watched Dr. Montgomery—with the extraordinary help of others—save the life of a woman who was in desperate need of a kidney. "He did it!" Valen exclaimed, excitedly.

The next time I found myself traveling south on I-83 was three weeks later, as six of us relaxed in a large, late-model minivan headed for Dr. Montgomery's cocktail party. Bill drove the spacious six-seater Honda that he'd borrowed from Gene Garrod. Rounding out the party-going group were Kris, Noah, Valen, myself, and Pam. Pam hates social gatherings of this sort. Normally, wild horses could not drag her to a party like this. She admitted she is more comfortable with her animals, such as her Hungarian Vizsla dog, Zsa Zsa. So it was a minor miracle that we convinced her to come along.

The party was held in the downtown Baltimore residential loft of Dr. Montgomery, on Fountain Street, with a fabulous view of boats in the harbor across the street. We knew we had arrived at the right place when we spotted the Ford Shelby Cobra.

Once inside the funky second-storey loft, we were met by Dr. Montgomery, who was nattily dressed in a black Nehru jacket with matching pants. Bill, Noah, and I wore business suits. Our respective partners were also dressed to the nines. Kris looked elegant in a three-piece chocolate brown chiffon outfit that featured beaded trim on the hems of her jacket, sleeveless top, and skirt. Valen was exquisite in a sequin-covered baby-blue dress with dainty shoulder straps. Her fashionable upswept hairdo with cascading curls was a definite Cosmo look. She sported a pair of dangling gold earrings and a matching necklace.

All five of us—and we weren't alone in our opinion—agreed that the belle of the ball was Pamela K. Cover. She will be embarrassed by this description, but she was stunning in an ultra-stylish, bluish-grey dress accented by a wide silk cummerbund around her small waist. Her waist-length brown hair with a reddish tint was worn up, with thin locks that fell delicately over her forehead and on the sides, cascading past her ears.

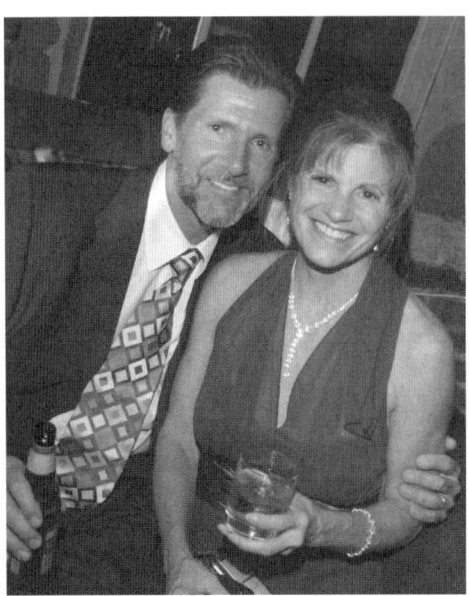

Valen says her parents have never been happier. The camera doesn't lie!
Photo by Maximilian Franz

The large, renovated loft was furnished in an eclectic mix of "oh my gosh!" items that ranged from a stuffed lion at the top of the stairway, to the authentic reclaimed brick walls and wood flooring. An oversized wooden century door suspended from the ceiling served as a table. Guests gathered around the unique table to sample a cornucopia of tasty morsels, including caviar, aged cheeses, assorted fruit, and other meaty delicacies and seafood. A half-dozen uniformed caterers roamed the room throughout the evening offering a variety of hors d'oeuvres and drinks.

A few thousand bright red rose petals had been strewn on the wood floor for this occasion that was attended by members of Dr. Montgomery's staff, his two children, some former transplant donors and recipients and their spouses, and other elite members of Baltimore society. I met a gentleman who is a speechwriter for senators in Washington, DC, and is also a transplant donor. J.P., as he is known, took me behind the well-stocked bar and pulled out a few bottles of a special beer he had brought back from a recent trip to Argentina. It is Quilmes, and I found it to be a lovely, golden, pale lager with a nice taste of hops. I looked for it upon my return to Toronto and discovered it was not available in the city's beer or liquor stores. It was my only disappointment following the cocktail party adventure.

The party was billed as an evening of celebration to recognize the establishment of The Margery K. and Thomas Pozefsky

Professorship in Kidney Transplant Surgery. Margery is an acclaimed potter and former kidney recipient. Her husband, Tom, is an internist on the Johns Hopkins faculty. Many years ago, Tom wanted to donate a kidney to his wife, but their blood types were not compatible. At the time, Margery asked if they could swap with another couple, but physicians told her there was no nurse co-coordinator to arrange that, so she donated money to hire a nurse manager. Margery received a kidney from her son, Kenneth Payton, on October 13, 2000, and is doing well.

As Chief of the Division of Transplantation at Johns Hopkins Medicine, the doctor and host of the event had a few special highlights planned for the evening. And there was one very memorable and spontaneous event that involved Valen.

Earlier that day, Dr. Montgomery had hired a crane and operator to lift a grand piano onto the second-floor exterior, roofless, rear ledge of his loft. Workers then moved the heavy and delicate musical instrument inside the condo and placed it at the far end of the room. When someone asked him about it, he reached into his pocket, pulled out his camera phone and showed us photos of the entire operation.

The piano was a backdrop for one of the evening's highlights: a recital by Denyce Graves. Ninety minutes after the five p.m. start of the party, everyone moved to the far end of the room to listen to a half dozen songs performed by the woman who has rendered her musical talents at The White House and who was named *Glamour* magazine's 1997 Woman of the Year.

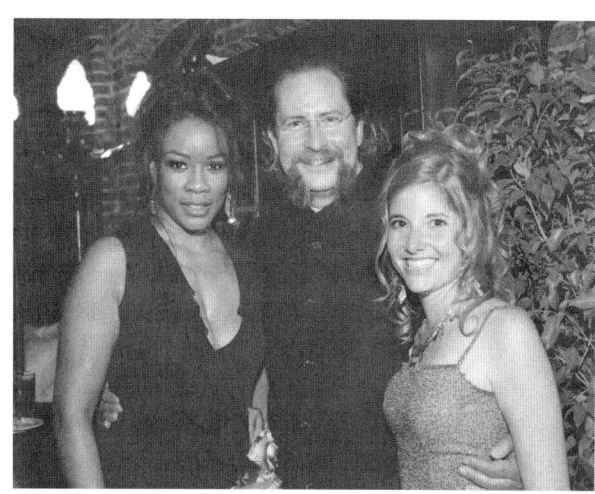

Opera singer Denyce Graves, Dr. Montgomery, and Valen.
Photo by Maximilian Franz

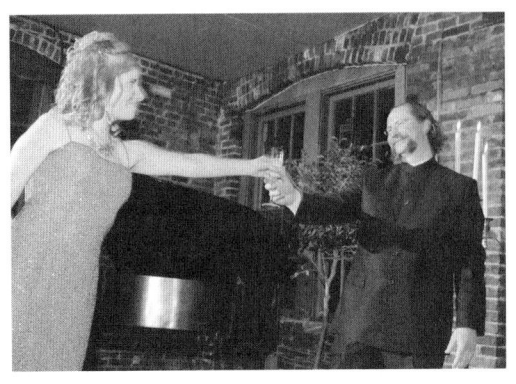

Valen hands a glass of wine to Dr. Montgomery so he may toast his guests.

Photo by Maximilian Franz

We listened in rapt attention to the woman of the evening, who received a bouquet of flowers from her companion and party host at the end of her recital. When the extensive applause died down, Dr. Montgomery stood to the left of the piano and made a few welcoming remarks. He introduced the guests of honor and spoke of Margery's dream of reaching out to people who are in need of kidney transplants but who have no hope and nowhere to go. Now, thanks to her generosity and the dedication of countless professionals at Johns Hopkins, glimmers of hope can be transformed into the miracle of transplantation through paired donation and the incompatible transplant program.

When he ended his informal speech, Dr. Montgomery called for a toast in honor of Margery and Tom. As we all raised our respective drinks, Dr. Montgomery looked a bit perplexed. The coolheaded, steady-handed physician looked at the table next to him that held a massive chocolate cake in the form of the famous, green-colored Johns Hopkins Dome, but he did not see what he was looking for. He shrugged, looked at the gathering of friends and said: "I don't have a glass of wine. How can I make a toast?"

Without missing a beat, Valen, who was standing a few feet from me, strode across the rose-petalled floor and handed him her glass of wine. She turned on her gold-colored, open-toed shoes to return to her place next to Noah, when the doctor called her back. Nonplussed and a little startled by the invitation, Valen retraced her steps and stood at his side, facing the crowd. He placed his left arm around her shoulder and brought her close to him. "This is Valen Cover, a former patient of mine," he proudly announced to the hushed gathering. "When I first met Valen, she was a very, very sick girl. I did not think she would survive." He spoke passionately and compassionately about how the gift of a human organ can change a person's life, and he talked of Valen's courageous struggle with PKD and other illnesses and how she had recaptured her life.

Both he and Valen were unprepared for this spontaneous moment. So were a lot of others. I thrust my glass of Buenos Aires Quilmes beer into the hand of the closest person to me—Noah Keefer—while I fumbled in my pocket for my digital camera, notepad, and pen. I held my camera at arm's length and could see in the viewfinder that Valen was crying. I glanced to my left and spotted Kris standing by a nearby window. She, too, was wiping away tears.

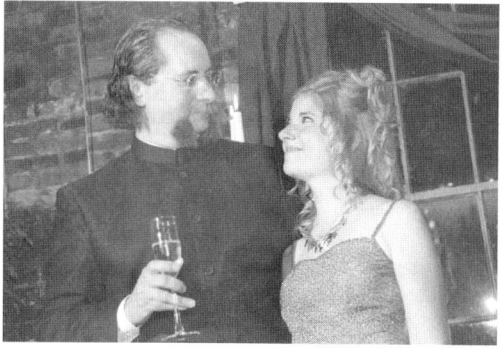

I snapped pictures and scribbled comments as I heard them. "For me, Valen crystallizes the wonder of living. To see her here tonight, so radiant and beautiful, reminds me what I do for a living and why I do it. She will be part of my spirit forever."

When the party resumed, the unlikely heroine of the night was swamped with good wishes. One prominent guest congratulated her for getting

Valen becomes teary-eyed when Dr. Montgomery makes an impromptu speech in praise of his former patient.
Photo by Maximilian Franz

up in front of everyone "because that's what this professorship in transplant surgery needs to hear—a story like yours." Brigitte Reeb, one of the doctor's staff members, told Valen she is an inspiration to people like her who work in the transplantation field of medicine.

We left later that night, each with a gift bag containing several items, including bottles of wine (Luna di Luna Cabernet/Merlot) and two of Denyce Graves's CDs, *Memorial* and *A Cathedral Christmas*.

Weeks later, I asked Valen what the evening meant to her. She said it was a turning point in her life, and Dr. Montgomery's remarks about her represented a crucial moment. "When he introduced me to all of his friends and colleagues,

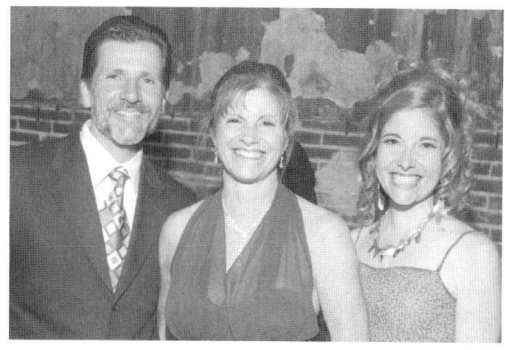

Valen is seen at the October 21 cocktail party with two of the most important people in the world, to her.
Photo by Maximilian Franz

it was by far one of the most rewarding moments of my life and it meant so much to me that my parents were there to hear it," she said. "The emotion, bliss, and gratitude that I experienced that night was humbling. I have never been so honored."

Valen revealed that ever since her transplant in 2002, she has had a desire to work in the field of transplantation. "On that evening, in Dr. Montgomery's unique loft apartment, I felt a calling to do even more with my life. I have immersed myself in volunteer work with the PKD Foundation ever since my transplant, but I became firmly convinced at that cocktail party that working in some capacity in the field of transplantation is where I belong. This is my passion. I believe that I beat the odds for a reason; and that is to do meaningful work in society and to help make a difference."

Valen would not have to wait long to see her favorite transplant surgeon at a social event again.

Four weeks after attending the lofty cocktail party, Valen found herself at a high-society ball at the Hyatt Regency Baltimore. She had been invited by Dr. Montgomery as his guest to sit at one of two tables reserved in his name. The occasion was the 22nd Annual Gift of Life Gala sponsored by the National Kidney Foundation. The event honored Dr. Montgomery, who was presented with the Champion of Hope Award for his innovative approaches to expanding live donor renal transplantation.

Valen and Noah arrived at the November 17th ball in their finest threads; Noah was a dashing figure in a formal tuxedo, and Valen wore a floor-length, taupe gown with attached train. An elegant flower pattern was evident throughout the smooth, silky material. Thin dress straps crisscrossed her back and along the shoulder blades, exposing her back and scoliosis scar. Accessories included a matching shawl and a purse that hung from her shoulder and dropped to her waist. Her teardrop earrings featured a taupe stone surrounded by diamonds. Her hair was French-braided up the back with curls on top and bangs dropping softly down the sides of her face. The heels of her shoes were clear and the tops adorned with a shimmering, sparkling material. The footwear was not glass like Cinderella's.

The Saturday evening gala was billed as a commemoration of the state of Maryland "from the mountains to the shore and everywhere in between," and the night included a silent auction, cocktail reception, dinner, and dancing to the sounds of New Monopoly. When Master of Ceremonies Fred Manfra announced the presentation of the Champion of Hope award to Dr. Montgomery, the renowned doctor approached the podium and accepted it on behalf of the many people who have worked with him to bring the miracle of kidney transplantation to patients who have been left behind by the transplant community.

In his acceptance speech, he spoke of the appropriateness of the name of the award, because most of the hard-to-match patients his team cares for in

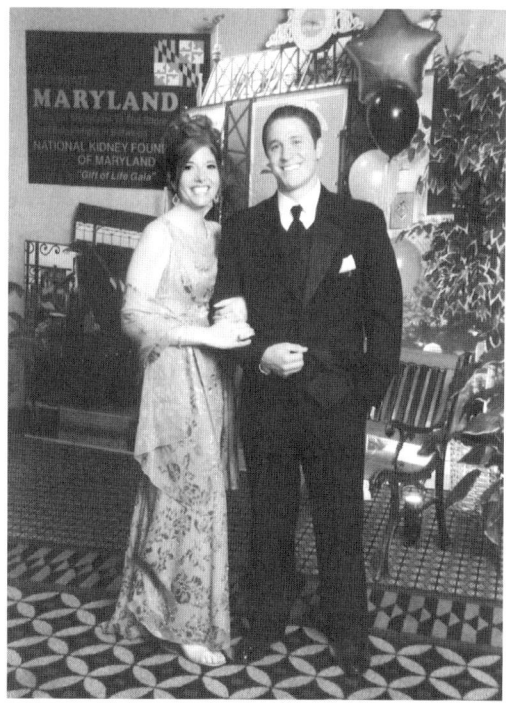

Valen and Noah attend the National Kidney Foundation of Maryland "Gift of Life Gala" November 2007.

the incompatible program have been told there would be no hope of their ever receiving a transplant again. He informed the gathering that some of his patients had been tethered to a dialysis machine for twenty or thirty years and had become progressively sicker and more despondent. "They come to Hopkins from all over the country in search of restoration and hope." The audience heard that nearly 300 of these patients have received the gift of life at Hopkins through incompatible transplantation and paired kidney donation.

In his entertaining and informative speech, Dr. Montgomery said he remembers each of his patients, and some were in the audience. "Many have become like family," he said, as he told the stories of several people who had come to him devoid of all hope for life or even a better life. He spoke of a young girl from Shamrock, Texas, who had raised money from bake sales, bull roasts, and country dances to be able to travel to Baltimore's famous hospital. He talked of a fifty-year-old gentleman from Kentucky whose previous four transplants had all failed after less than a year. And he plucked everyone's heartstrings when he told the story of a twenty-five-year-old woman whom he evaluated several months previously and who had already lost three transplants and had run out of blood vessels for dialysis. Tragically, she died the day after Dr. Montgomery met her. "We didn't have the opportunity to help her," he said, with sadness in his voice.

He spoke of the difficulties he faces in terms of creating innovative techniques and procedures and plans for transplantation, mostly because many hospitals are becoming disinclined to take on these difficult and costly cases. "It takes courage to offer hope," he said. "I am privileged to work at an institution filled with courageous people."

He did not mention Valen by name but as he spoke his eyes scanned the room. Occasionally his gaze would fall on his prized former patient sitting at his table in the taupe evening gown. And when their eyes locked, Valen always had a ready smile for her champion of hope.

11

The Ex-Marine

Friends I have had both old and young,
And ale we drank and songs we sung.
— *Charles Henry Webb*

I have never heard Valen sing a song, and I've seen her drink beer on only two occasions. Both times she sipped a Corona with the ubiquitous lime stabbed onto the rim of the bottle. So I can't say if she sings with friends while drinking ale, but I do know she has more friends than a brewer in a small town on a hot summer day.

She has many friends her own age and a few pals twice her age. I am proud to say she regards me as a close friend, too. I have seen her interact with people of all ages and both sexes, but she seems to have a magnet in her heart for men in their fifties and sixties. I have talked to her about this, and she admitted that part of it could be the influence that her former neighbor, Walter Smith, had on her during her childhood. Valen's father agreed, saying Walter was such a kind old man who helped to lay the groundwork for the love and respect for older gentlemen whom she chooses to befriend today. T.S. Eliot called men like us the "quiet-voiced elders."

I related a story to Valen one day about a lesson taught to me by Andrew Atkinson, my nineteen-year-old nephew who attends the University of Guelph, west of Toronto. He and I were driving to his grandfather's house — my wife's father. Andrew thought it was pretty cool that the nephew and "Uncle Dennis" were going to spend the day with his granddad and take him to lunch. I wanted to let Andrew know how much I admired the eighty-eight-year-old patriarch of the family who lived alone in a Guelph condo. "You know, Andrew," I said, "I can talk to your grandfather about any topic under the sun. He reads the *Toronto Star* every day, cover to cover, and keeps up with current events on the TV news. We can talk sports, politics, religion — you name it — and we can have a great discussion about anything."

I sensed that Andrew was impressed. He turned down the car radio to hear more.

"In fact," I continued, "If he weren't eighty-eight years old, he and I would probably be good friends and hang out together."

Andrew turned in his seat, gave me a sympathetic stare, and cut me down like a big oak tree: "Dennis, you should never put an age restriction on friendship."

He was right. I was chastened. When I relayed the story to Valen, she used a two-word affirmative that she and Noah like to employ when they want to act silly and pompous. "I concur."

One of Valen's closest male buddies was Ed Loch, a colleague at Lincoln General's 300-person, three-storey head office on York's Concord Road where the two worked. I can't explain the special bond these two had except to paraphrase French author Montaigne and say no more than "It was because he was he, and she was she." Ed was most impressed with what he called her "doggedness" in the face of her disease, and he truly believed she would have made a great Marine. He liked that she was not part of the self-centered "Me" generation and admired that she was the exact opposite, displaying a maturity and wisdom far beyond her years. He referred to her as "Wonder Woman" and a role model to many who know her. He believed the mark of a person is how he or she deals with adversity, and this Marine of twenty-six years who had gone where thunder sounded many times in his military career, had his young friend marked as a survivor of the highest order.

Some people just have a kind and gentle heart that comforts friends, and many people clearly saw this in Valen and Ed. The two met for lunch almost every Friday, sometimes at Charlie Brown's Steakhouse for a salad, or often they'd go for sushi at a local Japanese restaurant, Masa. Ed would offer his fatherly advice to Valen on everything from her social life to encouraging her to go back to school and get a college education, to his remarks on the meds she was taking. He called her "girly-girl" and he loved to give her guidance. "Hey girly-girl," he once said when she was struggling with a problem. "You either take the high road or you take the low road. Me? I always take the high road."

Valen, in turn, would lend a sympathetic ear as Ed listed the various medical procedures he had undergone that particular week.

Often they would set their past and present ailments aside and just be silly. One Friday, at El Rodeo, Ed ordered a chili relleno that was spiked with extra-spicy seeds that made him break out in a sweat. He said Valen kept handing him napkins to wipe the sweat from his perspiring brow, and with each batch of napkins she passed to him, the more she would giggle, until they ended up in a fit of giggles. Moments like this were a good respite for both the former and current patient, so they could forget their physical ailments for a brief time.

Valen looked forward to these weekly chinwags, but truth be told, it was Ed whose chin did most of the wagging. It was widely known that when Ed spoke, you never ran out of things to listen to. My Canadian East Coast farming relatives had an affectionate expression for people like Ed: "He could talk the ear off a cornstalk!" Often, the conversation was a monologue by Ed, as he would talk of his hypoglycemic shock, or that his temperature had dipped the previous night and his blood sugar was down to an alarming number. He spoke of the many blood transfusions he was getting, or how the tumors in his pancreas were progressing. He was not complaining. It was like an educational seminar. When he counseled colleagues and friends who were suffering with cancer — which he did often — he was helpful but abrupt: "You got it. Deal with it!"

When I asked Valen to describe her friendship with the man who was nearly a quarter-century older than her, she said people mean a lot to her, and he is one of many. "We can learn a lot if we just sit and listen," she explained. "Ed talked a hell of a lot and I listened a lot. He was a tough ex-Marine but he needed someone like me — someone besides his family — to listen and understand what he was going through. He made me feel like I was helping him, especially in his final days. It was difficult for me, because I didn't know how many more lunches I would have with him. I always looked forward to them."

As a veteran of far too many operations and infirmities to count, Valen was a great listener. She knew the square root: Been there. Done that. Who could ask for a better friend than one who comforts us in our afflictions? Despite the difference in their ages, they comforted each other to the end.

Ed died on Monday, July 30th, 2007, at Johns Hopkins Hospital in Baltimore. He was fifty.

I met the former United States Marine Corps (USMC) master gunnery sergeant for the first time just a dozen weeks before he made his last salute on earth. I traveled to his hometown of York in one of my roles as a contract editor for *Kingsway News*, a quarterly sixteen-page newsletter for the 2,900 Canadian and American employees of Kingsway Financial of Mississauga, Ontario. The company Ed worked for, Lincoln General Insurance, is one of Kingsway Financial's thirteen subsidiary companies. I wanted to introduce this remarkable man to my readers, and Ed, who was on disability leave, was motivated by a wish to send a clear message to his colleagues in both countries to take care of their health. He had cancer eighteen months before he was diagnosed and wanted to send a warning to others to be "aggressive" with their health; get checkups; do research; know things when you visit your doctor; know your body; and ask your doctor questions. Moments after meeting him and turning on my mini-tape recorder in a human resources meeting room on the first floor of the company's head office, Ed was firing off his wish list for others. He looked at me intently through rimless glasses and occasionally stroked a slightly graying moustache and goatee when he spoke. "Get a burial policy before you get sick, and pay it off. Get at least $500,000 Term Life Insurance." He was speaking in staccato sentences as though time were of the essence. We both knew it was.

I used two ninety-minute tapes on the recorder that day, even taping as he strolled through the office, talking to his fellow office workers; accepting sympathetic greetings; and dispensing advice. "I believe in taking care of people and I want that to be my legacy," he said. "In all aspects of your daily life, you've got to care about the people — including, and especially, the people you work with." I took photos with my Canon SD600 digital camera throughout the day, including one with three colleagues in his Special Investigation Unit (SIU) Department; and another of Ed standing at attention in front of the head office building.

My favorite picture of the day was shot as I walked behind Ed and Valen along a second-floor hallway. We had visited Valen in her Claims Department office area, and she took some time away from her duties to accompany me and Ed to other areas of the building. I was walking behind them and captured a heart-rending scene of Valen striding slowly with her weakened friend. Her arm was around his waist and he was holding onto her. She appeared tiny and vulnerable, yet she was the picture of strength. In contrast, her tall and lanky friend, wearing blue denim jeans and a blue, long-sleeved shirt, looked like a lean cowboy walking into the sunset. I watched the native of Wichita Falls, Texas, from my rear position and I thought of an old saying that "brave men rejoice in adversity and brave soldiers triumph in war." As I raised my camera and saw in my viewfinder a man sauntering down a long hallway, slowly, but tall and erect, and true to form, it was evident that he was facing his final battle with courage, faith, true grit, determination, and a continuing desire to help others.

My interview with Ed continued that evening when Valen met us at York's Harp & Fiddle Restaurant for shepherd's pie. Valen sipped on a soda while the Marine and I enjoyed one of Pennsylvania's famous Yuengling Traditional Lagers from "America's Oldest Brewery" in Pottsville. I knew Ed was becoming weary. He'd been answering my questions all day, and there was more information I wanted to extract, but we kept the conversation light at first. The previous week, Ed and his wife, Fran, had taken what he called "some lizard time" in Key West, Florida, attending the tenth anniversary of the FBI National Academy (he's a graduate). My wife and I had spent a few days in Jimmy Buffet's "Margaritaville" just two weeks

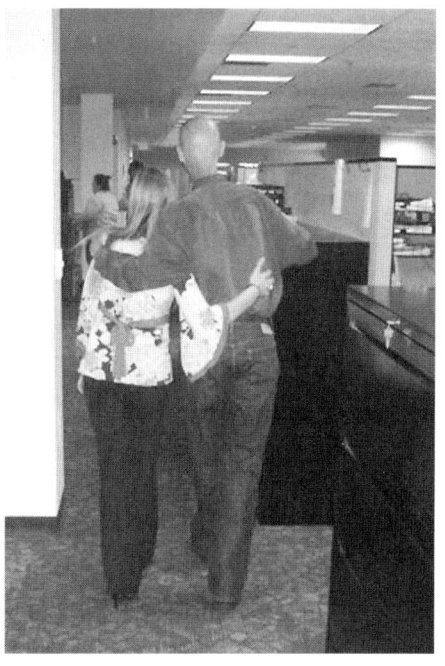

Valen and Ed take a stroll down a hallway at Lincoln General's Head Office, three months before his death.

before that, so we shot the breeze about our favorite places in the most southern tip of Florida, especially the bars on Duval Street like Sloppy Joe's and Fat Tuesday. We agreed the number one bar is Capt. Tony's on Greene Street. My favored spot in this southern-most community of continental USA, just ninety miles from Cuba, is Hemingway House. Ed revealed that his "favorite place on earth" is Mallory Square in Key West at sunset.

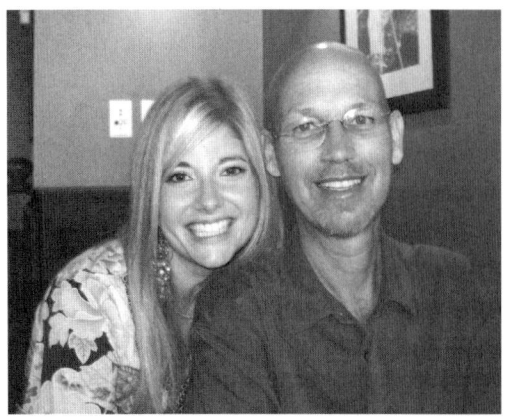

Author Dennis McCloskey took this picture of Valen and Ed Loch at York's Harp & Fiddle Restaurant.

Valen was very silent during the meal, respectfully sensing that this was still "work," and my interview with Ed was not over. Ed barely touched his dinner as he chatted about many things that evening; about his eighteen-year-old son Connor and how Ed wanted to live long enough to see him graduate from high school in June. I heard about Ed's backyard koi pond that's dotted with lily pads, and he shared with us his admiration for the fictional character Don Quixote. I asked if he felt like a knight in shining armor. "Maybe. I seem to want to help people and fix things for them before helping myself. And like me, Don Quixote jousted at windmills. I see him as a man who always tried despite the odds and who took up causes and challenges that others felt could not be surmounted. But at least he'd try. Yah, I guess I've always seen myself as Don Quixote."

I regarded this as my opportunity to fire off one last "interview" question. "If Don Quixote is your favorite fictional figure, name three people who inspire you most."

He thought for a moment. Drained what was left of his Yuengling and placed the mug on the table. "My father, for one."

He stared at the empty glass. "My boss, Tim Kirk. He is an extraordinary leader. The man could herd cats."

"One more," I coached.

"Valen."

There was a slight pause. Valen looked up. The clatter and chatter in the bar continued. So did Ed. "I am highly motivated by Valen and her battle with PKD. She is one of the few people who know the pain I have endured and who can comfort me on a level that no one else can."

Valen's lips quivered. Her eyes reddened. Ed reached across the table and squeezed her slightly shaking hand. She blinked back tears. She mouthed a feeble but heartfelt "thank you."

Ed withdrew his hand, wiped away a stray tear, and reached into the left pocket of his jeans. He retrieved two round objects about one and one-half inches in diameter. He placed one in front of Valen and one next to my now-empty beer vessel. "For you guys."

It was a replica medal of the United States Marine Corps. On one side at the top of the red and blue, golden-edged medallion are two words that represent the Latin motto of the USMC: *Semper Fidelis*, "Always Faithful." In the center is the insignia of a master gunnery sergeant. On the opposite side of the heavy, acrylic-covered facsimile of a military medal is the USMC logo with a golden eagle, wings spread, standing atop the world globe that is penetrated by an anchor. A banner flies from the eagle's beak. It reads: "*Semper Fidelis*." Ed always finished his e-mails with a five-word ending: "Semper Fi and God Bless."

Valen rubbed her fingers delicately on the surface of the souvenir medal. "I will keep it in my purse. Always."

Valen had arranged to have her mom, dad, and Noah join us for drinks and to meet me and Ed for the first time. When they arrived at around seven p.m., it marked the official end of our "work" day. A fresh round of drinks was brought to the table. The men opted for a strawberry beer that proved to be a zesty, fruity surprise for the palate that blended well with the wheat beer. The women drank sodas.

It didn't take long for the Pennsylvanians to start picking good-naturedly on the lone Canadian. I was outnumbered five to one, and it didn't help that I seemed to say "aboot" instead of "about" and ended far too many sentences with "eh?" Bill fired the best shot of the evening when he noticed I was playing with the medal, flicking it back and forth on the table from my right index finger to my left. As it slid on the glassy surface of the table for the umpteenth time, Bill wound up and fired a zinger my way. "Hey, Dennis. It's not a hockey puck."

Later in the evening, after another Yuengling, I said to no one in particular that I was having so much fun I'll have to suck on a lemon to wipe the smile off my face when I get back home the next day. Bill laughed and said he'd always think of me as his "lemon-sucking Canadian friend."

Around nine p.m., Ed was feeling the effects of the chemotherapy session he'd had the previous day, and my incessant questions over the past eight hours had undoubtedly tired him. He called his wife, Fran, to come get him. Twenty minutes later, she pulled up in front of the Harp & Fiddle. Ed said his goodbyes. It was the last time I would ever see him.

Over the next two months, Ed and I e-mailed each other constantly. "Just got a CT scan today and have to get a transfusion tonight at the hospital as my blood counts are very low," he wrote one day. "It's always something." That last remark was a favorite of his and it was coined by a comedienne we both admired: Gilda Radner (aka Roseanne Rosannadanna) of *Saturday Night Live* fame, whose book *It's Always Something* served as her memoir and her struggle with ovarian cancer. She died in 1989 at age forty-two.

"Hope springs eternal in the human breast" is another of our favorite quotes, and Ed was constantly full of hope, both for himself and others afflicted with illness. He befriended my sister-in-law, Ann Atkinson, who was suffering from pancreatic cancer at the same time. He e-mailed her constantly, offering advice and commiserating with her about the medications they were taking. When she would go to the family cabin on weekends and he wouldn't hear from her, I'd get an e-mail from Ed. "Is Ann okay? Haven't heard from her in a few days. Tell her to call or e-mail me any time. I hope I can help her. She has the right attitude about dealing with this stuff. She is in my prayers."

He seemed to have taken a shine to my family, but I am sure everyone he knew thought the same. When I told him that my wife and I were planning a week-long trip to central Pennsylvania at the end of August, he said he would take us on a tour of the battlefields of Gettysburg. And when he learned that my father-in-law, Bob, was a World War II veteran, he gave me a book to pass along to him, titled *The Spirit of Semper Fidelis: Reflections from the Bottom of an Old Tin Cup*. Bob read and loved the book, and as he learned more about Ed, through me, a feeling of mutual admiration developed between the two former soldiers. My father-in-law especially liked the line in Ret. Major Richard T. Spooner's book in which he quoted Shanghai Pooley as saying: "No one is really dead until he is forgotten." On April 8, 2007, I received an e-mail from the ex-master gunnery sergeant: "Tell Bob that I would come to attention if I ever met him. His generation—no matter the rank—are the true heroes of the world and far too many do not appreciate that."

Ed looked forward to his Friday lunches with Valen so much because weekdays were lonely for him when his wife was at work and his son at school. "I have a bit of the blues today," he wrote, right after I returned from my May trip to York. "I have to get up and start doing something, like clean the house and be thankful that I'm not taking the dirt nap." He reminded me that the illness was taking its toll on him and it was becoming harder to deal with it every day. "But I primarily distract myself by being involved and helping other people with their problems." On May 12th, his e-mail was brief. "Thanks for sending the pictures. Valen looks great. Can't say the same about me. Got an e-mail from Ann so no worries, we are in touch. Have to run to the store to get a shirt for Connor's suit for the prom tonight."

Ed received a lot of love and care from his family, relatives, and friends. If Valen was his lunchtime listener, I was his nighttime listener. One night he told me about three clinical trials for which he might be a candidate at Johns Hopkins Hospital. He called it a last resort. On May 25th, an after-dinner e-mail informed me of his latest decision. "I have decided when I can no longer do chemotherapy I am not going to do the Johns Hopkins thing. I don't want to try and suck the last drop of juice out of my life. I just want to go out with a sense of dignity."

I talked to Valen and she said not to worry. "Ed's not a quitter. He'll be okay."

In a way, she was right. He attended Connor's graduation on June 8th from Central York High School and it was a shining moment for the proud father as a thunderstorm raged outside the auditorium. But high winds, a deluge of rain, rolling thunder, and lightning did not dampen his spirits, especially when Connor was recognized among the top five percent of the graduating class of 323 students. He also received several academic awards. "It was a good night," he reported the next day. "I thanked God last night that He let me make it to see the ceremony."

Ten days later, the roller coaster took another dip. He went to breakfast with his family for Father's Day. But he was sick afterwards and wound up spending the rest of the day in bed. "Oh, well, at least I was here for Father's Day," he wrote. Later, he and Valen would have similar stories to share. Valen, too, was with her immediate family and grandmother for Father's Day, but she experienced severe stomach cramps—so much so that she said it ruined their Father's Day dinner entirely.

Not long after, Ed sent me one of his longest and most promising e-mails ever. He was full of optimism. He had started on a new drug that raised his blood sugar, and he said he felt better than he had in the past three months. He was also starting a three-times-a-day injection of a drug that suppresses his insulin production, which was out of whack due to the large tumor on his pancreas. It was confirmed by two cancer doctors that he had a rare form of pancreatic cancer called insulinoma. He was going to be sent to a doctor at Johns Hopkins who specializes in that form of cancer and he was left with a sense that he might have more time left than he'd originally thought. "I am cautiously optimistic but I have a lot of questions before I jump on the good news bandwagon. If I have an extended life span it's strictly due to the power of prayer. So many people are praying for me, I'm sure God is tired of hearing about me." His spirits were further buoyed by the recent news that his married daughter was pregnant. He ended his e-mail with a request: "Keep those prayers coming. I could get to see my grandchild."

On July 5th, he was just as buoyant after meeting with yet more medical experts. "It's all very confusing but I am told that at a very minimum I have at least a year left from this month."

Valen arranged to meet Ed for lunch at a local restaurant on July 11th. It was a Wednesday. Not a Friday. Didn't matter. This was a special occasion. After careful consideration and consultation with Valen, I had decided to write her life story and publish the biography in a book titled *My Favorite American*. I was convinced that hers was such a compelling story, I couldn't *not* write it. I was being pulled from the inside and pushed from the outside, and we were both very excited about the project. She couldn't wait to break the news to Ed. Likewise, I was anxious to hear of his reaction.

I called her after lunch.

"So? What did he say?"

"I didn't tell him."

"What? Why not?"

"He wasn't feeling well. He had two blood transfusions yesterday and another is planned for later today." She sounded disheartened. "He was so down I did not have the heart to tell him our good news. Maybe you could tell him this evening. He might be feeling better."

I e-mailed Ed later that evening and outlined the details of the book, explaining that Valen would be the central character of the non-fiction book and PKD would be a major theme. I relayed Valen's altruistic comment that by reliving her dark, sickly days and telling her story, it might help and encourage others who are lacking hope and faith. I also asked him to reflect on his friendship with Valen, because when he was feeling better, I would like to interview him about their unique and special friendship.

I heard from him early the next morning. It was a brief e-mail message. He was on his way to the cancer clinic for another blood test. He said his red blood cell count was 5.9. It had never gone below 7.5 when he was undergoing chemotherapy treatment. He said the people at the test station said they had never talked to a patient whose blood count was that low and who was still conscious.

He ended the rushed note by saying he would write more about the book and my request for his input. "Suffice to say I'm in for whatever you want me to do. Looking forward to Gettysburg trip this August. Gotta run to cancer clinic. Semper Fi and God Bless."

It was the last time I heard from Ed.

He spent his remaining days in Johns Hopkins Hospital. When I hadn't heard from him the week after his last e-mail on July 12th, I asked Valen if everything was okay. She said she had talked to Connor and was informed that his dad was in the hospital "for some tests." She and I never had a chance to say goodbye to Ed, but maybe that's the way he wanted it. Earlier in July, he wrote to me saying: "I've had a great life and I have no regrets." What more can we ask?

A gathering of family, friends, and co-workers met at Heffner Funeral Chapel & Crematory on Kenneth Road in York on Friday, August 3rd, for a Celebration of Life Service at 5:00 p.m. I could not attend. My brother and his family were visiting from British Columbia, and we were at our log cabin, a two-hour drive north of Toronto. Ed loved sushi, so we had our own celebration of life in his honor. At 5:00 p.m., I hoisted a bottle of Rickards Red beer and sampled a rice, vinegar, seaweed, and smoked salmon sushi roll in his memory. What more could a friend do?

Ed is survived by his wife of twenty-five years, Fran, and three grown children: Erin, LaDonna, and Connor.

When Connor spotted Valen standing at the back of the room before the service at the funeral chapel, he approached her to ask if she had gone up to "see Dad." She said no, she wasn't sure if she was ready for that yet. He accompanied her to the open casket. Fran said to Valen: "Ed would want me to ask how you are doing." Valen was taken aback. "I should be asking how *you* are doing."

As she stood before her departed friend, Valen sobbed her heartfelt concern that she had lost her guardian angel. "I'll help fill that role," Connor said quietly.

Tim Kirk (the "cat herder") delivered the eulogy for his friend and colleague.

An on-line guest book was posted on the Lincoln General internal Web site that was visited by scores of friends and co-workers who wrote poignant messages. Brian Makowski wrote of Ed's positive attitude and outlook on life, and Patricia Eline said he was an inspiration to all. Donna Shirley called him a true hero, and Lincoln General's then-president and CEO John Clark commented on Ed's "discipline, knowledge, humor, integrity, passion, and his loyalty to all those he loved and respected and who loved and respected him." He also wrote: "You meet people every day but you only meet a few that teach you lifelong lessons. Ed, thank you for teaching us how to live our lives."

Another on-line guest book was posted by the local newspaper, *The York Daily Record*. Among the thirty-five messages from people in California, Florida, Colorado, Nevada, New Jersey, and Texas, several were from Marines in Okinawa, Japan. "The example of grace and dignity in the face of his own mortality is something I will always remember," wrote Bob Bratton of Jacksonville, North Carolina.

The message I posted noted that his legacy will be the way he took care of people around him. I added a final salute to a fine man and exemplary ex-Marine and ended with his signature sign-off: Semper Fi and God Bless.

When I first wrote about Ed in the June 2007 edition of my Kingsway newsletter, he was pleased with the three-page article and photo spread. I titled the story "Man on a Mission." The next time I wrote about him was in the September issue. The heading over my obituary of Ed Loch was titled, "Mission Accomplished."

I was concerned about how Valen would react to her friend's death. Kris and I were soon relieved to learn that she was being stoic and strong. In an e-mail to Kris two days after the service, she said she misses him so much. "You would have liked him a lot. He chewed my ear off and lectured me (in a good way). I will miss our weekly lunches."

Ten days later, she reassured me in much the same manner. "I miss him terribly but I don't dwell on things over which I have no control," she told me on the morning of Wednesday, August 15th. "I accept things that I cannot control and I appreciate the good that comes out of them. Ed's spirit lives on because he has given a little piece of himself to so many people. I believe he is spread throughout the world."

Later that afternoon, Ed was buried with military honors in Arlington National Cemetery. Valen was in attendance, having driven to the nation's capital with colleagues. She was dressed patriotically in Ed's honor. She wore navy-blue dress slacks, a red blazer, white short-sleeved blouse, red pointy high heels, and red jewelry. Her hair was styled in a French twist with hairclips shaped like blue stars.

What more could a friend do?

12

The Motorcycle Accident

*"On the occasion of every accident that befalls you,
inquire what power you have for turning it to use."*
— *Epictetus 55 AD–135 AD*

On Wednesday, May 30, 2007 — two months to the day before
he died in a Baltimore hospital room — Ed Loch sent an e-mail to
Valen at 11:33 a.m. asking if she would like to "do lunch on Friday."
It was a typical message to his young friend and confidante. The
salutation was a familiar one: "Hey there, girly-girl!"

His morning e-mail brought her up to speed on his struggle
with hypoglycemia and low sugar levels. Despite his physical ailments, Ed was in an upbeat mood. His daughter, Erin, and her husband, Todd, had visited on Sunday and they feasted on crabs and
corn. On Monday, Ed's friend, Mike Hodge, dropped by. Mike, who
had lost both legs in the Vietnam War, owns an all-black, three-
wheel Harley-Davidson motorcycle. He takes part in the annual
Rolling Thunder motorcycle ride each year and he had just arrived
in Pennsylvania after a continent-wide ride on his H-D from Washington State. Rolling Thunder is a non-profit organization of over
eighty chapters in the U.S. and abroad and is comprised mostly of
men and women who are veterans from all wars and peacetime. Ed
regarded his friend as an inspiration. Ed's chatty note ended with
his trademark, "Semper Fi. God Bless." He then left to pick up his
son, Connor, at Central York High School, a brand-new school of
1,500 students.

Ed would have no way of knowing that Valen was attending an
off-site business luncheon with her bosses and would not receive
his e-mail for two weeks. As he backed out of his driveway at 1899
Brandywine Lane, he knew he would be early to pick up his son.
It usually took him about thirteen minutes to travel the five-mile
distance to the school at 601 Mundis Mill Road. Normally he was

late picking up his son. But on this auspicious day, he expected he would be early.

I, too, was unaware of Valen's meeting away from the office. Inexplicably, I felt uneasy because I had not heard from her in a week. At 12:54 p.m. on May 30th, I sent a brief e-mail asking if everything was okay. Judging by the time and subject heading, I must have been in a hurry, because I take pride in punctuation, grammar and proper spelling; but this time the title read: "How r u?" The text read: "Hey Valen, when I don't hear from my little girl in over five days, I start to wonder if all is okay. Is all okay?"

I knew she had recently been in the hospital with an infection, but I tried not to reveal any sense of foreboding or apprehension. So, I kept the message light: "I hope you are well and you enjoyed the Memorial Day long weekend and that it was a happy, hair-raising, hilarious, high-spirited, harmonious, honkin' . . . ah, what the 'H,' I hope it was a helluva good weekend!"

As it turned out, all was not okay!

At 12:52 p.m.—two minutes before I pressed the "send" key from the computer in my home office in Canada—Valen Elizabeth Cover was lying on the rock-hard asphalt surface of the eastbound lane of Mundis Mill Road in the middle of the intersection at North Sherman Street in York, Pennsylvania. The motorcycle on which she had been riding lay next to her. The damaged heap of metal was deader than Elvis.

Mere moments before a two-ton vehicle came crashing down on her, Valen was riding on the back of a 2006 Dyna Wide Glide Harley-Davidson. The motorcycle driver was her boss at the time and a family friend, Bob Galloway. The pair was returning from the luncheon meeting to the Lincoln General head office on Concord Road. Days later, Valen would recall that she had been enjoying what she termed the "feel of freeness" as the wind swept through her long hair that fell below her shoulders. The sun had provided a warm glow on her face. Her freedom ride ended when a twenty-two-year-old woman, driving a brown 2007 Toyota Corolla, slammed into the back of Bob's motorcycle at thirty-five miles per hour. The bike was stopped at a red light. The front middle of the car struck the bike with such a force that the heavy 1440cc Harley was thrust into the center of the intersection. Bob was thrown from the machine and lay unconscious on the road.

The state of Pennsylvania does not require motorcycle riders to wear a helmet. The sixty-year-old resident of Limerick, Pennsylvania, was not wearing a helmet on this ominous afternoon. Valen was, but it was a half-helmet style, without a Department of Transportation designation. It flew off her head as she was propelled backwards from the Harley, over the backrest and into the air. She landed with a sickening thud on the metal front hood of the car. As the vehicle swerved to the left, the sound of now-screeching brakes filled the air. Valen was thrown to the road near the disabled motorcycle and its owner. She crash-landed on her tailbone a second before her head and left elbow smashed into the pavement.

A woman travelling behind the Toyota witnessed the accident. She would tell the first police officer on the scene, William Pouzzotto of Springettsbury Township Police, that she was facing a "steady red light" when the car in front of her struck the motorcycle. The officer would note on his Commonwealth of Pennsylvania Police Crash Reporting form that the daylight, rear-end collision occurred on a dry road in no adverse weather conditions. He issued a traffic citation to the Toyota driver, on the scene.

There was another witness to the accident.

A man was also stopped at the same intersection, facing the motorcycle and the Toyota. He was jolted out of a calm and oblivious moment when, to his horror, he caught the unbelievable sight of two people flying through the air. He slammed his transmission into Park, grabbed his cell phone, bolted from his small truck, and called 911.

The man was Ed Loch.

The ex-Marine and Lincoln General employee rushed to the accident scene and was preparing to put his military-trained first-aid knowledge to its test when he stopped in his tracks. He was stunned to realize he knew both victims. "Oh my God, it's Valen!" he exclaimed to no one in particular. "And Bob Galloway!" Ed would tell me a few hours later in a phone conversation that it was a bizarre and surreal experience.

Three months later, on August 30th, Kris and I visited the scene of the horrific accident with Valen, now recovered. We walked along the wide boulevard and paused at the sparsely traveled intersection. I faced the direction the vehicles would have been traveling and was struck by the obvious visibility of two large traffic lights suspended on a horizontal aluminum pole that spans the width of the lane. On the left is a farmer's field that ends at a thick cluster of trees. To the right are spacious lawns of emerald-green grass. It is a rural setting on the edge of the city. Clear and unobstructed visibility is evident from every angle: north, south, east, and west.

On her return visit to the scene, Valen was animated—initially—as she recounted the events of that grim day. I snapped photos of the accident site and the victim. Valen was dressed in a pair of fashionably torn and faded hip-hugger jeans, a goldenrod-yellow top, and a pair of double-strap sandals that accented her brightly-painted, crimson-red toenails. I snapped photos while Kris taped Valen's vivid recollection of the collision and its aftermath: "We were stopped at the red light, and the next thing I knew, I was flying in the air, backwards. The bike was pushed to the middle of the intersection, and as the car swerved diagonally, I was thrown to the ground and landed in front of the bike. I might have blacked out for a minute but when I woke up I clearly saw Ed on his cell phone in front of his truck. I looked back and saw Bob lying next to the bike. He was completely still. I heard Ed talking on the phone about the accident. It was crazy and it was surreal. It felt as though I were in a movie, watching how I was going to die. I thought I *was* dying, because Ed was there and he had no earthly reason to be there. Then I thought: 'He is my guardian angel and he is here to protect me and I am going to be okay.' My faith told me that God spared me again."

When Valen becomes excited, she speaks very fast. By now, Valen was talking a mile-a-minute. She was wearing a pair of trendy, large-sized, black-rimmed sunglasses so I could not see her eyes. She paused and took a breath. "Oh, look," she exclaimed in child-like wonder. "There's another butterfly. I love butterflies!" The temptation to ask if she had butterflies in her stomach was too obvious and inane, so I suppressed the question. She continued: "I saw the car. It was crunched up in the front and a liquid was leaking on the ground. When I realized I was lying in the middle of the intersection I panicked because the first instinct, when you're lying in the middle of an intersection, is to get the hell out of there. I went into shock because I started to scurry on my hands and knees toward the side of the road. Ed was telling me not to move, but I was so shocked and confused, I just had to get to the side of the road. That's when I started to feel the pain. I felt the side of my head and it felt squishy. I freaked out. I pushed on it and it was soft and swollen. It was a contusion, and the swelling was about two inches from the normal surface of my head. I kept pushing on it and Ed told me to stop but I was so afraid I had a blood clot."

Soon, Valen heard the sound of sirens. She was sitting on the side of the road. Ed was holding her hand. He had attended to Bob, who had regained consciousness and was now in a sitting position. He appeared to be suffering from a head injury and severe "road rash." Valen held on tightly to Ed's hand telling him over and over again that he was her guardian angel. She told him "a million times" that she loved him; that she was scared; and that she would never ride a motorcycle again. "I told him I loved him because I thought if I am dying I want someone to know that I love them," she said. She had felt it was her final day on earth, but she was lucid enough to tell Ed she needed her purse. It was back at the office and she needed her "two o'clock meds." There was something else in her purse, and though no one spoke of it until I brought it up weeks later, the thought of it might have entered her subconscious mind and provided a flicker of light in her cloudy brain: the replica medal of the United States Marine Corps that Ed gave her at the Harp & Fiddle Irish Pub, twenty-three days earlier. The one she said she would keep in her purse. Always.

The firefighters were the first emergency crew to arrive, and one began to administer first aid to Valen. She was afraid she would pass out or have a seizure, so she tried to tell him that she'd had a seizure disorder in the past and has had a kidney transplant. "I said: 'I am not normal.'" She grinned at the recollection of that comment. I could not tell if her eyes were smiling behind the contemporary shades. "I was super dizzy and my head was spinning. He told me to lay flat on my back. I am big on eyes. If I am not well, I focus on someone's eyes and I get strength from that. I looked into his eyes and for some reason I liked him. He held my hand as I lay there. I was in pain but he made me feel comfortable. When he tried to get up and leave to do something else, I would not let him go. I knew he had to look after the other people but I wanted him to stay with me. I felt good while he was with me. I wouldn't let him leave until I was in the ambulance."

Before we left the scene of the May 30th mishap, Valen said she wanted to sit on the side of the road in the same spot and face the same direction she had on the day of the accident. Kris and I left Valen alone with her thoughts, but her demeanor spoke volumes. It was a poignant scene. Her glasses rested on the crown of her head and her left eye was partly closed, almost in a wince. Her left leg was curled under her right leg. One hand rested lightly on the pavement but she grasped the lower portion of her left leg with the kind of tight and firm grip that a local firefighter must have felt ninety days earlier.

Valen and Bob were taken by ambulance to York Hospital. The driver of the car was not injured. The car and motorcycle were hauled away by Louie's Towing Service and transported to its location on Industrial Highway. Valen asked Ed not to call any of her family members. She did not want to worry them, especially her mother. But she soon changed her mind.

Some people do not believe in accidents. There are only encounters in history, they say. Some people do not believe in coincidence. Valen is one of them. "Everything happens for a reason," she often says. Now, as she lay battered, bruised, and bleeding in York Hospital, she thanked God she was alive but she wondered why. "I don't feel sad," she mused while sitting on the side of the road three months later. "Sometimes I cannot fathom what my body has been through and I'm still kicking. This is just one more awful thing I have endured in my life. It's kind of crazy."

Valen believes that Ed's appearance at the scene was no accident. She called it a "spiritual event." I agreed with her. I have always believed that coincidence is nothing more or nothing less than a spiritual occurrence. Ed, himself, told me the day after the incident that God put him there. "Normally I am late picking up my son at the high school, and yesterday I was early. I'm glad I was there to help whoever it might have been, but for it to be Valen and Bob, well, that's truly a miracle." Even strangers who hear of the synchronism say it has a touch of otherworldliness. My nephew, Andrew—who told me to never place an age restriction on friendship—did not call it bizarre or weird, the kind of language I might expect from a teenager. He said it was "a divine appointment."

Whatever it was—a chance event or a freak encounter—Valen and Bob knew they'd been in an unfortunate calamity that would amaze and confound them for a long time to come. Thankfully, Bob was treated and released from the hospital the same day, having suffered minor external injuries, including a head wound, bruises, and a great deal of soreness.

It was a different story for Valen.

She was wheeled into the emergency room of the 466-bed community teaching hospital on South George Street and was soon being treated for a variety of ailments: she had cuts on her foot and knee; a bruised hand and crushed ring finger; massive swelling and bruising on her lower back that was diagnosed as a large hematoma, or a swelling filled with blood. She also had hematomas on both sides of her head—the swelling on the left side was larger than the right—and she suffered a massive concussion. In addition, her back and neck were stiff and extremely sore. A bruise the color of a purple eggplant appeared on her pelvis. Doctors were especially concerned about the condition of her kidney and the Harrington rods in her back.

Ed had called Valen's father to inform him of the accident, but Ed had very little information to impart other than she was alive and coherent. Bill works in Harrisburg, twenty-three miles from York. He immediately called his wife, who could reach the hospital before him. And she did. Pam rushed to her daughter's side, arriving before any other family member. Valen was lying on the hospital bed still in a daze and feeling groggy as medical staff scurried about, preparing her for a CAT scan on her damaged head and performing a series of other tests. Doctors worried that her vulnerable, donated kidney could have been damaged when she landed on the pavement, so an ultrasound of her kidney was ordered.

In the middle of this organized confusion, Pam walked into Room 341. Valen immediately became calm. "I felt instantly relaxed as soon as I saw her," she would tell me later. "It was like an angel walked into my room. I said: 'Oh my God! There's my mom!' I was so thankful to see her; so thankful to be alive. I will always remember seeing Mom that day and how she looked and how I felt." Soon her father arrived, as did her brother Brandon, whom she had not seen in awhile. There had been some family strife that had concerned Valen. Ever the peacemaker, she had stopped at his workplace the previous day, to see him. "If something really bad had happened that day, it made me happy knowing that I had seen him the day before."

With her family by her side, doctors and nurses worked feverishly on their patient. Blood was detected in her urine, so cultures were sent to the lab. Doctors started her on an antibiotic due to a low-grade fever. Noah, whom she had met just two months before, rushed to her side. Subsequently, he visited her every night after getting off work and sometimes stayed until two a.m. She felt so much better when he was with her in the hospital. And he never complained of being tired, saying it was what he had to do every day. "He was awesome," she said with a wide smile. "Physically, I felt weak, but when I looked at him, I felt strong. He was so wonderful in my time of need." The day after the accident, Ed brought her flowers and a charger for her pink cell phone, the one that plays a few notes from the Guns N' Roses song "Patience" as its ringtone. Ed immediately recognized that she was "shaking and scared by the pain" as she relived every agonizing moment that followed the collision. Kris and I were preparing to drive nine hours to see our little "wounded dear" but Pam suggested it was not such a good idea. "Keep in touch with her by phone," she counseled. "Your visit will be much more rewarding when Valen is herself again." Mother knows best. We followed her advice.

York Hospital is the region's leader in advanced specialty care. Its 3,400 employees serve a population of 520,000 in south central Pennsylvania, and it has been named a top-100 hospital in the nation six times in a row. Valen was in good hands. With her injuries slowly healing, doctors released her from the hospital after a week. Divorced from her husband in March 2007, after a marriage that had lasted just over two years, Valen was still living in their apartment in nearby Red Lion. But now her new temporary home would be her parents' house on Susquehanna Trail.

Again, she was in good hands.

But she was not out of the woods. Not by a long shot. Not physically, and certainly not mentally.

The two-week period that followed would be what Valen described as "the lowest point ever, in my entire life!" This from a person who has already endured unimaginable pain and suffering in her young life. "I was not myself," she conceded, almost apologetically. "I was a mess!" She was desperately trying to deal with the physical agony of recovering from her injuries as well as the loss of some hair from both sides of her head. Doctors believe the reason for the hair loss was a combination of the swelling from her head injury and the stress and trauma she had suffered as a result of the concussion.

When she lost her hair, Valen lost her spirit. Her mother called it the straw that broke the camel's back. "Our normal Valen is very depressed and angry," Pam told me ten days after the accident. "She is thankful that she survived the accident, but she is quite tired and weary of everything. She is so down on herself. She just wants to be like every other twenty-four-year-old." Her next statement saddened me even further. "Mentally, it is going to be a rough road back for our Valen." Even Ed was confounded by Valen's depression. "It's odd," he lamented. "It's the first time I have seen this side of Valen. Poor thing. She is making progress but she gets frustrated."

I felt a range of emotions as I contemplated the motorcycle spill from my home north of the U.S. border and I thanked God that Bob and Valen were given the gift of life. I was elated that our "fallen angel" had been spared once again. I told Ed in an e-mail that it must be for a reason: "I think God has favorites and she's one of His darlings. She seems to be living life from one miracle to another. God has a plan for her. I just know it. I can feel it. All she has to do is figure out what it is and fulfill it. God keeps handing her lemons. She just has to keep making new batches of lemonade."

In my heart, I feel The Plan has something to do with helping to find a cure for PKD.

I called Valen often when she was in the hospital and while she was recuperating at home. Each time I heard her weak voice I felt I was listening to the voice of an angel. Sometimes I cheered her; sometimes she cheered me. She told me I should write a book about her and call it *Nine Lives.* It was the afflicted comforting the comforter! When she was well enough to go online at her parents' house, I e-mailed her a steady stream of positive messages. She loves music—she had taken piano lessons in her youth until illness forced her to stop—so, on the morning of June 12th, less than two weeks after the mishap, I told her about a new CD by Canadian songstress Avril Lavigne. One of the songs is titled "Keep Holding On," and I told Valen the words seemed written expressly for her: "Stay strong . . . you'll get through this . . . I'm here for you."

Later that day, I was listening to Detroit singer/songwriter Bob Seger on my iPod while walking through the ravine behind our home in Richmond Hill. I told her I thought of her as he belted out his blue collar themed song, "No More." The words resonated in my mind as I thought of the hardship Valen had endured in her short lifetime. I understood why she was depressed. The sound of Seger, a rock icon of the ages accompanied by his Silver Bullet Band, wailed mournfully and painfully from my iPod: *"Well, I don't want this / No, I don't want this / I have had enough—no more."*

Like Ed Loch, Valen is no quitter, but I felt so much compassion for her predicament and I wondered: *Why, Lord? Why do bad things happen to good people?* (A week later, I mailed Harold S. Kushner's book of a similar title to Valen.) I was delivered a gentle reminder as Seger continued singing: *"No one gets to walk between the rain."* I shared my thoughts—and Seger's words—with Valen and helped her to realize that she was not alone in her darkened space. "The world has teeth," I preached, borrowing a phrase from a Stephen King novel. "It can bite you anytime it wants." And it has. In fact it has taken quite a few chunks out of her mind and body. It has made a few meals out of her! I let her know it bites others, too, and I spoke of a friend who lost his wife that same week. On Sunday, Bob Burkett was sharing a few drinks and some laughs with his wife, Wendy, on the porch of their home. On Tuesday she died of a heart attack. I also reminded her of my sister-in-law, Ann, and her continuing struggle with cancer. No one gets to walk between the rain!

My "Seger" e-mail was a lengthy one. I included a story about visiting my cabin the previous weekend and nearly hitting a deer that leaped in front of my car on the secondary road that leads to my gravel driveway. The next morning, as I was leaving the cabin at dawn, the same deer—or one just like it—stood at the end of my driveway, as if awaiting my arrival. It did not move as I gingerly approached the stately doe in my new, silver-grey Honda Accord. The sound of gravel under the quartet of Michelins resonated in the early morning stillness. I stopped, practically brushing the deer's tan-colored hide. I rolled down the window and we made eye contact. Our eyes locked and we continued to stare at each other. She wasn't even startled by Seger's classic trademark song, "Like a Rock," which blared from my CD player. When I e-mailed Valen later that morning to relate this story, I joked that initially I thought the deer was apologizing for scaring the piss out of me the day before. Then, I knew the underlying meaning of our early morning meeting on the edge of the forest: "Valen is out of the woods," the deer appeared to be reassuring me. "She's going to be okay."

Valen assured me she didn't gag while reading my tale of the white-tailed deer. That afternoon, at 12:36 p.m. on June 12th, she sent me an e-mail from her parents' home where she was convalescing. I save all my e-mails (thousands are kept in computer file folders) but this one ranks among the Top 10 Hall of Fame e-mails that I have received. She wrote: "You are an amazing, amazing man! I just finished putting on my makeup and doing my hair to try to look pretty for the day and, well, that just all went to shit because I am sitting here crying! Thank you so much for this e-mail. You are a remarkable man and you have a way with words like no one else I know. You have surely touched my life like no other person."

Since I could not see my wounded little dear in person, I continued to jam her in-box with inspirational messages that let her know this, too, shall pass and she would soon leap higher and farther than ever. "Life is a grindstone and whether it grinds you down or polishes you up depends on what you're made of" is a quote by J. Thomas Holdcroft that cheered her up. I added that she is a diamond in the rough and she will always be a shining jewel in the eyes of many people. Hokey? Sure it is, but she said it made her smile.

My scrapbook artist wife created custom-designed cards for Valen and sent them to her by ground mail. I discovered a passage on the Internet by that famous author, "Anonymous," typed it on parchment paper with a tranquil beach scene as a background, and mailed it to her. When I visited her office three months later, I noticed it posted on her cubicle wall. It is titled "It's Going to Be Okay": "Just give things a little time. And in the meantime . . . keep believing in yourself; take the best care; try to put things in perspective; remember what's most important; don't forget that someone cares; search for the positive side; learn the lessons to be learned; and find your way through to the inner qualities . . . the strength, the smiles, the wisdom, and the optimistic outlook that are such special parts of you. It's going to be okay. I know it will be. Because I know you."

I wasn't the only friend to fill her mailbox with messages of encouragement, hope, and love. Of the multitude of well-wishes that Valen received during her dark days after the accident, a favorite of hers came from a co-worker, Monica Melendez, who told her in a June 6th e-mail how much she missed her. "Even though you are so small, there is no way you are going to let something like this bring you down. You are my hero! Get well soon and hurry back. We miss you!"

Two days after the crash, I had received so many e-mails asking about and commenting on Valen, I decided to read them to her in an attempt to lift her spirits. I called her hospital room on the sunny day of June 2nd and asked Valen if it was a good time to read some messages I had received. "Sure," she murmured. "I'm not going anywhere." I carried my portable phone outside, sat on the front porch, told her to fluff her pillow, sit back, and enjoy. We talked for thirty minutes. I relayed telephone messages I had received, asking about her, but most of the time was spent reading letters from my friends, colleagues, neighbors, and relatives who had heard of the unfortunate collision. "Life can be cruel. She is so young," wrote my friend Shirley DesRivieres from Sarnia, Ontario. "Thank God Ed was there for her. It was no coincidence. It was meant to be." Rich Henquinet, an assistant vice-president at American Country Insurance in Elk Grove, Illinois, wrote that his heart goes out to Valen and her parents. He informed me that flowers had been sent to Valen's hospital room that morning from "her friends" at American Country.

"Who's Rich Henquinet?" Valen asked from her hospital bed 400 miles away.

"A colleague of mine."

"I just got the biggest bouquet of flowers in my life. What a sweet guy!"

The then-president and CEO of her company, John Clark, wrote from his Chicago-area head office that he was devastated by the news of the accident and he and fellow employees were praying for the complete and quick recovery of this "incredible person."

"Aw, that's so sweet." I could hear the smile in her soft, angelic voice.

There were more. Lots more. From people who had never met Valen Cover. Just heard about her or saw her photo.

"Valen is so beautiful inside and out," wrote Nancy Carnahan of Kingsway General Insurance Company, in Mississauga, Ontario. "Whenever I have a bad day, I think of the story you wrote about her in our company newsletter and I am thankful that my problems are so small. You have to write a book about her."

From my best friend, Jim Mitchell, international president of Steelcase in Strasbourg, France: "Dennis, it is obvious that you are touched by this remarkable woman in many ways. You speak of her spirit in a powerful manner. Valen is full of grace and that is her strength."

"What a beautiful and lovely girl," from my sister Margie in Brooklin, Ontario.

And this, on June 1st, from neighbor Wendy Kosmachuk: "Dennis: I am so sorry to hear about your 'daughter.' We pray that her injuries are fixable and she is already on the mend. Does she know how lucky she is to have you and Kris as friends? You should write a book about her!" Moments after I read this message to Valen, Wendy drove past in her GMC Yukon SUV. She came to a stop, turned down the driver's side window and shouted: "How's Valen?"

"Talking to her right now."

"Give her my love."

Uzma Ahmad is a Muslim who worked as a senior internal auditor for Kingsway Financial in Mississauga. She has worked with Valen on a special assignment at the York head office. She wrote: "What horrible news. Sometimes we need to ask God why He would send such trials and tribulations to someone like Valen who has suffered so much. I am praying for Valen and may God give her comfort and peace to her family."

One of my favorite notes in the aftermath of Bob's and Valen's misfortune came from one of my special friends, Viviam Maria Lopez, of Miami. She's my favorite Cuban-American! I have known and admired the talents of this vibrant and youthful woman since 1999. We e-mail often and see each other far too infrequently. On the morning of May 23rd—seven days before the crash on Mundis Mill Road—Viviam sent me an e-mail, commenting on nothing more than our special platonic relationship. "I cherish and rejoice in our friendship so much," she wrote. "No words or situations could ever come between the special bond that we continually share. It can only get better and stronger with time. This comes straight from my heart."

By day, Viviam works as executive assistant to Roberto Espin, president of Hamilton Risk Management Company. Every Monday evening, the vivacious and talented Viviam hosts a two-hour program on Miami radio station "Serious Jazz" 88.9FM WDNA. Her show is called *Fusion Latina*. She plays Latin Jazz music from Cuba and elsewhere in Latin America, and has a worldwide audience, thanks to the Internet. That's how I listen to her program, and see her on the studio web cam. On the Monday after the accident, Viviam played a special tribute to Valen, Bob Galloway, and Ed Loch, "three special people who are not well tonight." At 9:27 p.m., Kris and I heard Viviam play *Keep the Faith* in their honor. She told me the next day that she had wanted to play a special song to their "health and well being; something that was upbeat, with a strong message, full of faith and confidence."

Later that week, I took a huge risk in an attempt to make Valen smile. I told her about a book I was reading, Stephen King's 1999 novel, *The Girl Who Loved Tom Gordon,* about nine-year-old Trish McFarland, who was lost in the woods. Valen has never asked "Why me, Lord?" even in light of all the troubles she has encountered, and I told her that is an admirable trait. Then I related a passage to her from King's book that tickled my black-humor funny bone. King was referring to the biblical character, Job: "When his life was ruined, his family killed, his farm destroyed, Job knelt down on the ground and yelled up to the heavens, 'Why, God? Why me?' and the thundering voice of God answered, 'There's just something about you that pisses me off.'"

Valen chuckled on the phone when she heard that. The next day she mentioned it in an e-mail to me. "The story you told me last night on the phone was funny. I think I probably do piss God off because I am so strong-willed, but I don't let the little obstacles that He throws at me stand in my way."

Valen appreciated the well-wishes from friends and co-workers and she said my dark humor lightened things up.

The upbeat missives may have temporarily dulled her period of despair, but did not wipe it out.

For the better part of June, Valen's mother took her fragile daughter to more doctors' appointments than either can recall. One week they went to a neuromuscular therapist on Wednesday; then spent seven hours on Thursday at Johns Hopkins Hospital for blood work, an ultrasound, and a visit with Valen's kidney doctor. Friday they were back at JH for another seven hours of appointments to see her dermatologist about her thinning hair and a skin cancer test. She also saw her internist, Dr. Mark Hughes, and others. The good news was that the two Harrington rods in Valen's back were still firmly in place and her kidney function was good; it had not been damaged in the fall from the motorcycle. The not-so-great news concerned her low blood count (she had lost a unit of blood due to the swelling and bruising in her back); neck and shoulder muscles that were tight due to the whiplash she suffered; and a low iron count.

Who could blame her for wallowing in despair? The American aphorist Mason Cooley wrote that hope and despair ignore one another's cries. Valen would sit on the porch of her parents' home and cry until her deep well of tear ducts could secrete no more. Amid the sobbing, Bill and Pam held out hope that the sadness would not last much longer. Their daughter was alive, and where there is life there is hope. They were confident she would climb out of this temporary abyss and reclaim her normal life, because they also knew there can be no mountains without valleys. This was another valley to ascend and another detour to maneuver. They suggested she see a psychiatrist, but Valen is self-assertive. She refused, claiming she did not need to see "a shrink." She is well aware of her strengths and she knows that tough times don't last but tough people do. She insisted she could deal with it in her own way and on her own terms. She has never taken anti-depressants, a decision backed by her parents and doctors, who agreed she was on enough medications.

"We were very concerned and we wondered how much more she could endure," Bill revealed to me months later in his living room, just steps away from the porch of tears. "The motorcycle accident was horrible and it could have been worse, but it took her out of a normal lifestyle that she was just beginning to create and enjoy. The accident was devastating to her. She couldn't work. She couldn't go out with her friends. She was hurt. Again."

Valen denies she felt sorry for herself during this dark period. "I was just not in a good place in my mind. I've never been like that, even during my worst illnesses." As she spoke, she rose from her chair, crossed the room and sat on the living room floor, legs crossed, facing her parents. "I was just so fed up," she continued, staring at the floor. "I just wanted to be like everybody else my age. People were telling me that I was lucky to be alive and to stop being so negative, and I knew they were one hundred percent correct, but they don't know my complex life. I was starting to enjoy life after my transplant and this shit happens."

I rarely see an angry Valen, but on this pleasant, end-of-summer evening, some of her suppressed anger began its slow rise to the surface.

"I just want to do so much, I can't sit still, and I have so much time to make up. I missed some prime time in my childhood because I was sick so often. When other kids my age were doing stupid stuff, I was fighting for my life! After the motorcycle accident, I just got into a shitty attitude and for two weeks I was not solidly myself. That's not like me. I couldn't even do my hair in the morning, so I started my day bawling my eyes out. Everything was just so overwhelming for me."

I wanted to ask how she overcame the glumness, but Valen was not finished. Her resentment was now palpable and her level of anger rising. "I look at so many people my age and I am sometimes very envious of what they have, but they disrespect themselves so much. It is so disappointing to me. I just want to shake them and tell them how good they have it."

"You can't tell someone that," her father interjected.

"I know. But I am so grateful and appreciative of everything when I'm healthy, and I try to enjoy life and I have the drive and ambition and desire to do so much. I just get angry when I keep having these setbacks."

The mood in the room, like the delicate flower sitting cross-legged on the floor, was now somber. "I feel like I am always a mess! That's just me. Always a mess! There's always something wrong with me. I hate that!"

Valen then revealed that she has learned to hide her illnesses. If she does not feel well, she does not tell anyone, so they won't be burdened by her afflictions. Sometimes she doesn't even tell her parents. She does not want them to worry that things will revert to the way they were before the transplant. "If I am not well, my parents go into this instant shutdown mood. I don't want to send Mom and Dad back to January 2002. I pray to God it could never get to that point again. It just can't. It can't get that ugly again! So, I often don't say anything to them if I am not well. I have had small problems since the transplant that I have not told them about. If it is necessary and they need to know, I will. If not, I try to get through it on my own."

I saw my opening. "Did you get through your depression on your own?"

Valen looked at her mom and they both smiled like only a mother and daughter could who've been through so much together. They had suffered a world of hurt, but could still grin through their tears.

"Mom got me through it. She snapped me out of my mood."

I had heard the story before, from Pam's perspective, and this was my opportunity to get Valen's take on her resurrection.

But first, this was her mother's interpretation in a late night e-mail to me in mid-June: "Valen's darkest moment was today at Johns Hopkins. We were walking down a hallway and Valen wore a blank stare. I motioned for her to follow me. We went into the rotunda of the Hopkins' administration building. At the back and along the side are three very old wooden telephone booths. I stood in front of one in particular. I told Valen that one dark day, when she was very ill, I went into one of the booths. I shut the door and I cried, because I did not think I could handle what God had put before me. I cried and cried until I could cry no more."

Pam's e-mail described her now-familiar story. She emerged from the phone booth, drained of tears and emotion, and walked around the corner of the grand dome of the building's main lobby. There she saw the towering statue of Jesus Christ and stopped to gaze at the carved, robed figure of marble, its head gently bowed and seemingly staring at her with such sympathetic eyes. Pam was frozen in time.

At the midnight hour in the stillness of her York home, with her dog, Zsa Zsa, by her side, Pam wrote: "I stood before Him, humbly, and said I would put all my trust in Him. And prayed that He would do what was best for Valen. As I told Valen of my deep pain, we both started to cry. We hugged and sobbed. She told me how lost she feels. How hopeless and helpless she feels. She told me how hard it was to go through the divorce. She talked of a fall she had taken at the beginning of the year when she severely injured her knee and had been frustrated at the slow healing process. Then the motorcycle accident. It was just all too much to bear."

Pam listened while her daughter talked in the shadow of the towering statue. It was a soul-cleansing and emotional event for both. "Somehow we regained our composure and continued our day. At dinner this evening, I saw a glimmer of hope in her eyes for the first time in weeks." She ended her letter the only way she knows: graciously. "Thank you, Dennis, for listening."

Valen echoed her mother's version of the moving event.

"Mom's right. It was my darkest time. I hated the loss of my hair. I hated everything. I was miserable. It wasn't like me, but I could not control it. Unfortunately, we lash out at the people we love, and I took my anger and frustration out on Mom. She had said something and I snapped at her. She gave me that hand thing that she does; the 'come here' finger. I walked toward her, grumbling and mumbling. She took me to the phone booth and described what happened. She said it was her lowest point. Then she took me to the statue. I was a mess. I was crying uncontrollably. The accident had saddened me terribly."

It was a turning point for Valen. Her mother discussed in a calm and easy manner all they had been through. "Mom stated that we have come so far and we have so much to be thankful for and that we can get through anything. She reminded me how awful things had been and that things weren't that bad right now and we are so lucky to be where we are today."

Valen was now baring her soul. "Mom basically told me to snap the hell out of it. She said some kind and gentle things and suddenly I felt grateful. I can't explain the feeling, but I stood there in front of that giant statue of Jesus, my eyes filling with tears, and I knew that I had not been kind to her and Dad. I apologized for not being very nice to her. I vowed, then and there, that I would put myself back together and make my parents proud of me. It was such a humbling moment, but I knew, instinctively, that I would get back on track, mentally."

Valen hesitated for the briefest of moments. No one interjected. This was Valen's time. In an instant, she collected her thoughts and continued speaking in a hushed, reverent tone.

"I am forever grateful for my wonderful parents. They are my strength. They have been with me through everything and they went through just as much hell as I did. It is hard for me to explain how much love and respect I have for them. I am often humbled by the amount of love we have for each other. I would not have survived without their care and their love." Valen looked up from her sitting position on the floor and asked a rhetorical question: "How do you thank someone who has devoted their life to you; given you everything? How do you repay such generosity and self-lessness?" She answered her own question by repeating an earlier heart's desire. "All I can hope is that I will make them proud of how I choose to live the rest of my life."

It's true what they say. Loving parents have caring children.

It would be trite to say at this point there wasn't a dry eye in the house. The atmosphere in the room was soulful. The only sound was the scrape, scrape, scraping sound of Zsa Zsa chewing on a large, cream-colored, rawhide bone.

Bill broke the silence. "Yah, she's back to normal now. She drinks beer!"

Corona to be exact. With a slice of lime.

Valen threw back her head and laughed. "I am medically allowed to have two or three drinks of alcohol a week," she said by way of explanation. "It's not bad for the kidneys. I never drank alcohol. Ever! And I have now decided to enjoy a beer once in awhile. Why not? Why can't I loosen up a little like everyone else? And start to enjoy myself and my life?"

I raised my bottle of Franziskaner German beer and toasted her with a familiar French-Canadian cheer: "*A votre santé*, Valen. To your health."

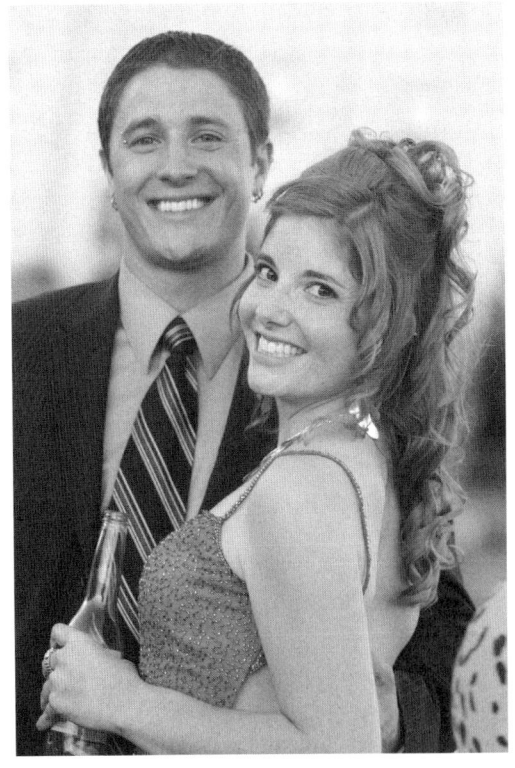

Enjoying a beer with Noah at the party in the doctor's trendy Baltimore loft.
Photo by Maximilian Franz

13

The Grateful Soul

*"Would anyone believe me if I told them that battling **PKD**
was the best thing that ever happened to me? Polycystic
kidney disease defines me. Rather than being bitter towards
life, I am loving life because of it."*
—*Valen Cover, in a letter to Dr. Montgomery,*
October 23, 2007

Valen was never as healthy or as happy as she was immediately after her kidney transplant. Five years later, she would tell me that when she woke up she felt "so freakin' alive it was ridiculous!" Her excitement was as clear now as it surely was in August 2002. "It was the first time I felt good," she said. "The first time I felt alive in a long time."

When she awoke from the transplant operation, she sat upright in bed and wanted to go for a walk. "I was so happy I could not shut up," she exclaimed. "My friend Adam Shaub was rubbing my forehead; my friend Emily was there with her sister, Rebekah, and my brother, Brandon, and of course my parents."

"Life was good again," said her relieved father when I interviewed him years later.

Mere days after being released from the hospital, Valen began recording her vital medical information in a daily journal, thus relieving her mother of the task. There was a significant difference in the serious tone of the chronicle of medications and the amounts taken, blood pressure, and food consumed. Two words and the ubiquitous Wal-Mart happy face filled an entire page in her first entry in mid-August: "AFTER KIDNEY." ☺

In the days that followed, the still-meticulous and detailed clinical data—as now recorded by the patient and not the caregiver—was interspersed by drawings of smiley faces. On September 5, 2002,

Valen studiously noted her blood pressure and pulse rate at 11:01 a.m. and added that she will "try and start beta-blocker tomorrow." Then she added: "First clinic appointment. Went great. GREAT DAY!! I can drive!" ☺

There were now plenty of reasons to smile in the Cover house. The physical scars were healing, but the emotional ones would take a little more time.

"Valen's illnesses and operations cost us plenty, but it wasn't so much a financial toll as it was an emotional one," Bill revealed to me. "That's where we hurt the most." To this day he admits to having "flashbacks" of some of the horrible events of the past associated with his daughter's illnesses. I boldly asked him to describe one of those flashbacks, and he complied without hesitation. "When her stomach was bleeding, the blood was clotting and forming into balls. Then her stomach would reject it and she would vomit the blood and choke on it. I would hold a dish under her mouth when she brought up those clots of blood and at times I would have to help bring them out of her mouth. I recall one time a nurse asked if I was okay with that because she had to leave the room to get help. I really thought it was the end when I was dealing with that. It was near Valen's nineteenth birthday. I can't get that out of my mind. There were also the times when she would come back from one of her surgeries and she didn't look anything like herself. I remember Pam and me just shaking our heads and wondering how the hell she had persevered, yet again!"

Valen, too, confessed that she suffers from occasional flashbacks, but they are normally associated with the motorcycle accident. They usually occur while driving, and especially when she's behind a motorcycle. She certainly hopes they will become less frequent as time motors on, but sometimes during the day she will experience an unpleasant flashback and relive a certain aspect of the collision or recovery period. "It can happen sporadically. It's not fun."

Bill and Pam paid a hefty price, emotionally, and it goes without saying that Valen paid dearly, physically. But her mental anguish was equally debilitating.

In one of my family discussions with the Covers, Valen conceded that her parents helped her overcome the mental and emotional aspects of her illnesses. "It would have been so lonely and sad to not have them there," she said. "I constantly looked into their eyes for strength and hope, and somehow I felt I was going to be okay because they were there."

Her father appreciates his daughter's gratitude but he does not accept the mantle of savior, exclusively. "She was able to see how important she was to other people. That inner awareness helped get her through a lot of difficult situations."

Valen thoughtfully digested this information and did not dismiss her father's opinion, but continued with her own mental concept of her survival.

"My parents wanted so much for me to get better; they altered their lifestyle just for me. I was only nineteen; I didn't have much in life, just them. If they had not been with me mentally and physically, I would not have gotten out of bed some days."

There was a measured hush in the room when I asked Bill what makes him proudest of his daughter, today.

He needed time to think about this. Like about a tenth of a second. "Without any doubt, it is her ability to persevere and triumph over everything she has endured to become a productive and happy and giving person who does not live a life of negativity and who does not dwell on the past. She lives for today and the future, and that makes me so proud of her."

It was a warm summer evening, but the comment caused a few chills and shivers among those present.

Bill noticed the quivering lips but continued: "It would be easy for her to become bitter about the entire ordeal she has been through but I haven't seen a moment of bitterness from her. She's had to deal with a tough life but she has turned it into a positive experience and dedicates a lot of her free time to helping others who are in similar circumstances. After all she has been through, all she can think of is helping others!"

While all the wet eyes in the house were drying, it gave me pause to consider what makes *me* so proud of Valen Elizabeth Cover.

If I had to sum up in one word all the myriad qualities I admire in Valen, that word would be "gratitude."

When Holocaust survivor Elie Wiesel accepted the Nobel Peace Prize on December 10, 1986, he spoke for everyone who has suffered intolerable pain when he said: "No one is as capable of gratitude as one who has emerged from the kingdom of darkness."

Valen would cringe to have her life compared with the annihilation of a million slaughtered Jews, and that's not what I'm doing, by any stretch of the imagination. I am saying that she is grateful for life itself—after living on the edge of darkness for so long—and she displays her thankfulness in many ways as she lives her daily life.

I have heard it said that gratitude is the most exquisite form of courtesy, and Valen is a very respectful young lady. "Gratitude is a fruit of great cultivation; you do not find it among gross people," Samuel Johnson wrote in the eighteenth century. It may be a rare commodity today in a world desensitized by technology, but it is as true now as it ever was. Valen is a classy young miss who displays gratitude to people, and that, in turn, makes her happy. French novelist Marcel Proust called people like her "the charming gardeners who make our souls blossom."

As my personal friendship and professional relationship with Valen blossomed, I became more and more aware of her appreciative nature. I'm not so naive as to think I am the only one on the receiving end of her thanks and praise. But I can attest to her quality of gratitude through her e-mails, cards, phone calls, and our visits that are too few and far between. On September 10, 2006—five days before my birthday—she gave me the gift of kindness when she wrote in an e-mail how much she appreciated my words of encouragement. "Your words empower me to feel stronger and to keep plugging away. You have such a way with your words that inspire me!" Wow! Me? Inspiring the inspirer?

Later that week, she ground-mailed a card to me. It was simply titled: "True Friends." Inside was a handwritten note: "Dennis: You have indeed made my life richer in so many ways! Thank you so much for taking an interest in my life battles and for taking the time to write to me and about me for others to learn from my experiences."

At Christmas she sent a card to her Canadian friend, mentor, biographer, unofficial stepfather, and northern neighbor. The cover shows penguins sliding down a snowy hill. She said she instantly thought of me when she saw the penguins all bundled up in toques and scarves. (Oh, I get it! It's cold in Canada but not in Pennsylvania? ☺) The card was addressed to Dennis ("Dad"), and she once again thanked me for the "kind, supportive, encouraging, and inspiring words of wisdom." She added this warm and flattering remark: "Your e-mails have brightened so many of my days! I am honored to be your friend." Then she wished me and my "lovely wife" a wonderful Christmas and a happy and healthy New Year before signing it: Valen ("daughter.") and adding the perpetual smiley face: ☺.

Her appreciation often extends to Kris, who makes customized cards for relatives, acquaintances, and friends like Valen. When Valen was hospitalized in 2007, Kris sent her a card decorated with a soft feather, an illustration of a stylish high-heeled shoe, and the words: "Wish Shoe Well." Another was an exclusive "Hang in There" card complete with a miniature wire coat hanger.

On July 31st—Kris's birthday—our grateful Pennsylvania friend wrote: "You and Kris are absolutely amazing! I don't know how I got so lucky and so blessed to have the two of you in my life. You two are so sweet and kind and I will never be able to thank you enough for all the thoughtful things you both continue to do for me."

Next on my list of VAQ's (Valen's Admirable Qualities) would be "kindness" and "courage," because she expresses incredible kindness toward people in trouble and immense courage in times of her own distress.

Benevolence seems to be second nature to her, and she performs acts of random kindness without fanfare. I was talking to her on the phone late one afternoon when she excused herself, saying she had to call someone in the hospital. A few days later, I remembered to ask her who was ill. I learned it was a woman who had undergone a kidney transplant operation a short while ago. Valen had not previously known her, but the sixty-something woman and her grown daughter had taken part in one of Valen's fundraising PKD walks. The daughter had contacted Valen to say her mother was fearful of the upcoming operation and would Valen consider calling her mother at home to reassure her that everything would be all right.

Valen did that, and more. She talked to the very sick lady on the phone for an hour to comfort her and explain there was nothing to worry about and that she should be excited because she was going to feel great after the transplant. Valen visited her in the dialysis unit and called twice more before the transplant. On the day of the transplant operation, Valen purchased "an awesome pot of artificial flowers" during her lunch break to bring to the woman after work. "I always wanted real flowers when I was in intensive care but I knew hospital rules forbid it after a transplant," she explained to me. "When I got to the hospital I convinced the nurse on duty to allow me to visit the woman in the ICU even though I was not a family member. The woman had had her transplant and she was sleeping off the drugs when I entered the room." It was an eye-opening experience for Valen to see the patient hooked to an IV bag, a tube in her mouth, and all the other paraphernalia that Valen knew had been attached to her own frail body following her transplant surgery. "I looked around the room and at the lady and I started to cry," she revealed. "That was me five years ago!"

It was early evening, and the family members had gone home, so Valen sat alone in the room with the slumbering woman for over an hour holding her hand. Just as Valen was putting on her coat to leave, the woman awoke, saw Valen, and began to cry. "She tried to speak, but she had a tube in her mouth, and I told her to save her energy and not to cry." A nurse entered the room, witnessed the emotion in the room and said she would remove the tube for a few minutes. When she did, the woman grasped Valen's hand and cried: "Thank you! Thank you!"

"Quit saying thank you!"

"Am I okay?"

"Yes, you are wonderful. And I think you are peeing!"

"Oh, thank God. And thank you!"

Valen loves the Helen Keller quote that she has adopted as a mantra ever since the motorcycle accident: "Life is an adventure or nothing at all."

And what was one of the first adventures Valen experienced following the May 30, 2007, accident? She had a beer for the first time. A Corona. With a twist of lime wedged onto the lip of the bottle.

Oh, and she climbed back on the horse.

Her mom loves four-legged animals, as does her daughter, but Valen also has a love for the two-wheeled beasts that her former pediatrician, Dr. Sean Campbell, calls "donor cycles." Although she has never owned a motorized bike, most of the men in her life are riders, including her father, her brother, and her partner, Noah Keefer. Less than two months before her motorcycle accident, Valen was planning to get a 2007 XL 1200 Harley Davidson Sportster Nightster. Her mother nixed the idea. "Mom got scared, and I backed out of the Harley deal,"Valen explained to me on April 4th. "She doesn't want me hurting myself."

I fully understood Valen's love for motorcycles the minute I saw the front license plate on her green Honda Acura. She and Kris were in Chico's buying each other a bracelet and ring. They were attracted by the inspirational words engraved on the heavy, silver costume jewelry they purchased, such as "faith, hope, peace, happiness, inspiration, spirit, love, and trust." The inscription on another piece they bought reads: "Respect, confidence, fairness, growth." While they shopped, I read *The New York Times* and sipped on a Caramel Frappuccino at the Starbucks next door. I glanced out the window of the upscale coffee shop and spotted Valen's car. I had never noticed her front license plate. I grabbed the only writing paper available—a Starbucks napkin—and walked to the car to write down the personal message: "LIV2RYD." As I was writing, Kris and Valen emerged from the store. As they approached the car, Valen smiled and shouted: "Hey, what're you doing, Napkin Boy?"

If Valen had a dollar for every time a relative, friend, or doctor told her that she should not be riding on the back of a motorcycle, she could probably buy a Starbucks franchise, or a Harley dealership! The objections were loudest in the weeks after the May 30th accident when she said she wanted to ride on the back of a motorcycle again.

I needed to hear this straight from the horse's mouth, so I called her one day to talk about it. I got her voice mail. I tried an hour later, and when she answered, she apologized, saying: "Sorry. I had to tinkle. My single kidney is doing the work of two." I told her not to apologize. "I'm just glad you can tinkle!"

When she confirmed her desire to ride on the back of a motorcycle again, I tried to dissuade her by telling her about a friend, Keith Dickson, who had been severely injured while riding his motorcycle in Wyoming not long after she had taken her disastrous spill. She was very sympathetic but took a pragmatic approach. "It's a tough decision to allow another's unfortunate accident to steer me from doing what I love to do," she rationalized. "If I focus on other people's misfortunes, I will miss out on enjoying my own life."

She is not blind to the dangers of motorized bike travel. "I know you can get severely hurt when a car hits you on a motorcycle, and I realize more and more how lucky I was to survive the accident. But at what point do I give up the things I enjoy in life, to be safe? Or, do I just put my life in the hands of God and fate and hope that my life will not be stripped away and shattered in a motorcycle accident?"

She paused and pondered the personal philosophy she had just expressed and asked another rhetorical question: "Who knows what lies on the road ahead?" She added that she loves the outdoors, and when she is riding on the back of a bike she is breathing life. "The sights I see from the back seat of a motorcycle are saved as beautiful snapshots in my memory."

On May 8, 2007, three weeks before her motorcycle accident, Valen sent me an e-mail and joked about being a "Harley Mamma." But she was not satisfied riding on the rear seat. "I have my motorcycle license and by the end of the summer I plan to get my own bike," she wrote. "I know they are dangerous and I'm sure if something bad would ever happen, it might stop me from riding again. But I love riding; it's my quiet time. My brother and I say we stay healthy because we're on bikes."

Ironically, something bad did happen, and during her convalescence, she admitted to me that it would be a tough decision to climb back onto a motorcycle again. But she did.

When she had recovered sufficiently, she convinced Noah to take her for a ride on his 1983 Kawasaki KZ 1100 Spectre/D. Afterwards she received flack from a few friends who felt she was tempting fate. But there was also understanding from those who believe that the threat of death makes some people more aware of their lives. Ed Loch believed she was pressing her luck. "As I was calming her on the side of the road right after the accident, she kept saying over and over that she would never again get on a motorcycle," Ed told me after her first post-accident ride. "She dodged a bullet. I knew she would get back on, but I hoped not." He also understood why she did it. "It's her life and there's a lot to be said about not letting bad things prevent you from living a full life."

In early 2008, I asked Valen why she wanted to ride on a bike again. Following are her comments about her first spin on a bike after she lay sprawled and injured on a York street.

I simply had to get "back on the horse" after the motorcycle accident. Noah and I went helmet shopping before the ride and we bought full-faced helmets. The only person I have ridden with since the accident is Noah. We rode to our favorite spot, which is a little place by the river at Yellow Breeches, north of Dillsburg, PA on Rt. 74. It's about 30 minutes from York. Noah suggested this location because it's a place we both enjoy together and I love to put my feet in the water. It was a fairly straight route with few turns and very light traffic.

Noah took his time and was so kind; he kept making sure I was okay. A few minutes after we left, he pulled to the side of the road, shut the motor off and got off the bike to make sure I was all right. After giving me a comforting hug, we continued our ride. I was very nervous. When we approached the first intersection, I tried to turn around even though I knew I couldn't because of the rods in my back. I was so afraid of what was behind us and what the other motorists were doing.

I experienced a lot of unpleasant flashbacks during the ride and kept looking over my shoulder. It was a challenge, but I like challenges. When we made it safely to our spot I got off the bike, removed my helmet, and let out a huge sigh of relief.

I wanted to do the ride because I was very frustrated and angry that the person who crashed into me took something away from me; something I loved with a passion, and it was turned into a tragic experience. After the accident, I was filled with so much anger every time I saw someone on a bike because of what happened to me. I wanted to face my fear and resentment and get back on a bike again. I'm glad I did. My head hurt and so did my back but it was worth it.

In the past, whenever it was a sunny day, I would want to do nothing else but get on a motorcycle. Unfortunately, it is just not the same now. I enjoyed riding so much, because it was like therapy and relaxation for me. I loved to feel the fresh air on my face, breathe it in deeply, and enjoy the scenery. After being in the hospital for so long, riding was like being in heaven.

I was frustrated and annoyed that the accident happened but I didn't want to let one experience stop me from continuing to do what I had once loved. It will just take time for the feeling of freedom and enjoyment that I experience on a bike to return.

I still have flashbacks of the accident when I'm driving. I had one on my way home from work today.

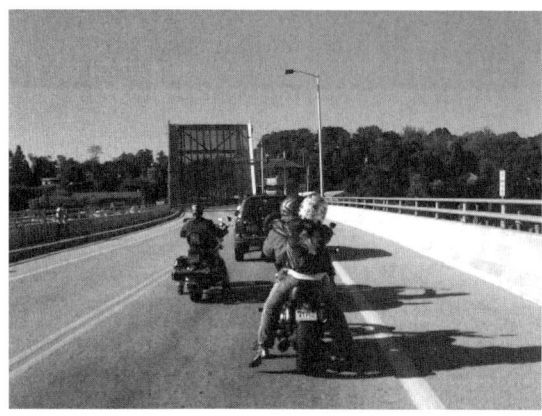

Valen hangs on to Noah on the back of his bike, waiting for the bridge to come down. They were on a group ride the autumn following Valen's May 2007 motorcycle accident.

"Sometimes there's just no way to hold back the river," wrote Paulo Coelho in *The Alchemist,* an enchanting and inspiring magical tale. And no one was going to hold back Valen Cover from doing what she enjoyed. Not after what she'd been through in the past.

There would be more rides after the initial post-mishap trip to the river. On Labor Day weekend, 2007, she climbed on the back of Noah's Kawasaki and they rode 123 miles in one day, to State College, Pennsylvania. They stayed overnight in the town of 38,420 and made the two hour and fifteen-minute trip home the next day. Later that fall, they joined her father, two of his work buddies, and family friend Bob Galloway as they rode their bikes on a day trip to view the brilliant autumn colors in rural Pennsylvania.

The rides were cathartic for Valen. She had triumphed over adversity once again and was regaining her confidence and enjoying a new zest in her life. Buoyed by her ability to conquer the dragons of fear, she sent me a quote that embodied her feelings. It's by Helen Keller: "Character cannot be developed in ease and quiet. Only through experience of trial and suffering can the soul be strengthened, ambition inspired, and success achieved."

It was onward and upward for Valen Cover.

Of all the defining moments in Valen's life—and there have been a multitude—one that stands out in her memory (and mine) is a second visit she made in the summer of 2007 to what the Covers call "The Jesus Statue."

She was acutely aware of her mother's initial visit to the Johns Hopkins phone booth when Pam was in the depths of despair, and fresh in her mind was the visitation with her mom after the accident when Pam displayed tough love and lectured her daughter about her attitude.

This time, though, Valen wished to make the pilgrimage to the statue on her own terms. Kris and I were honored to be with her when she did.

She wanted to spend time in the very same phone booth in which her mother sat when she had cried out for help. Valen also had a desire to meditate upon her life before the famous marble statue.

When we entered the administration building that houses the statue under the magnificent dome, we stopped first at the wooden phone booths. Valen entered, closed the folding door, and sat on a stool. Kris and I allowed her the private, quiet space she so hungered for. After an appropriate period of time, I gently rapped on the glass door and asked if I could take her picture. I heard the same polite and humble response that she gave when I asked to interview her for the first time nearly two years before. "Sure, if you want to."

The resulting photo is now one of my prized possessions. She is pictured sitting in the cramped phone booth, casting eyes heavenward. Later, she would tell me that she tried to imagine what her mother was thinking when a distraught Pam entered the booth for the first time. What is striking about the photo I took of Valen is that a bright light appears over her head. She and I know it's the flash from the camera, but some might suggest it represents the guiding light of Jesus who is leading her out of the darkness of past illnesses and into the light of a new tomorrow. Or, it could signify the shining light that Dr. Montgomery saw in her when he first met her. Valen called the appearance of the light "simply amazing" and suggested it could be a sign or an omen. I reminded her of Paulo Coelho's message in *The Alchemist* where he encourages all of us to follow the omens in order to find the treasure. "God has prepared a path for everyone to follow," he wrote. "You just have to read the omens that he left for you."

She rose from the hard, wooden stool and eased herself from the tiny compartment. We strolled the short distance to the rotunda, where Valen stood before the medical shrine, lost in her thoughts. She silently read the inscription written in capital letters on the pedestal of the statue: "Come unto me all ye that are weary and heavy laden and I will give you rest." Once again, Kris and I stood in the background, immersed in our own secret thoughts.

After a few reflective moments, Valen strode to one of the two guest books that are placed to the right and left of the statue on nearby stands by the entrance of the monumental room. I noticed that she was writing in one of the books, so I walked to the other bookstand. I wanted to read the very first message on the first page.

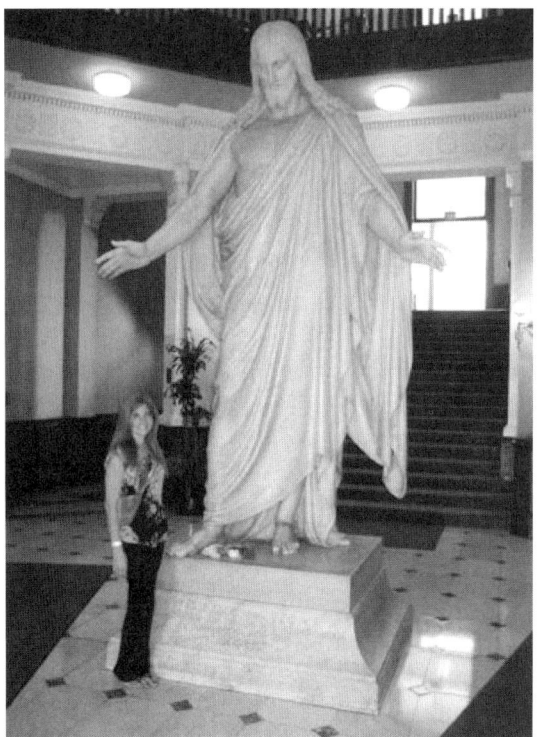

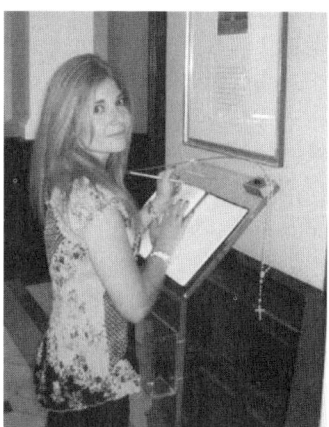

Valen writes a poignant message in the guestbook near the Jesus statue.

Valen visits the Jesus statue at Johns Hopkins in 2007 with Dennis and his wife, Kris.

An emotional visit to the Hopkins phone booth where her mother broke down several years earlier.

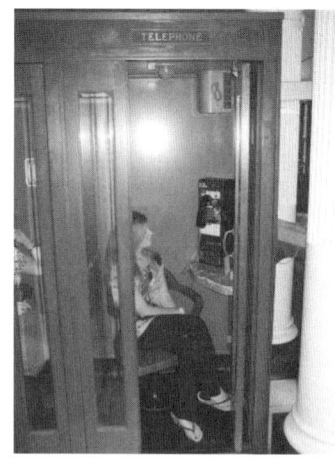

When all the pages are filled, the journals are stored in chronological order in Hopkins' pastoral care department. I read the message on page one. It was dated August 22, 2007, Kris and my thirty-second wedding anniversary. The scrawled note was a touching plea from a godmother regarding her sick godchild: "To who much is required, Lord, I don't ask for me, but for Rayla, my goddaughter. I ask that you touch her today and bring her out."

It was signed *"Valentine."*

I was struck by the similarity in names, so I walked briskly to where Valen was still standing to tell her about the coincidence. She was putting the final touches on her message and I could see she was crying, softly. I did not want to intrude but I quietly and respectfully asked if I could read what she wrote. She nodded her head and slowly walked away to join Kris. (She has also given me permission to reprint her words here.) This is what she wrote: "This is my first day at Johns Hopkins as a visitor, compared to what I am used to as being a patient. I am filled with such gratitude today that the tears won't stop. You know the life that I lived in Hopkins. Please give strength to all of the patients here like the strength you gave me so they, in turn, can enjoy life as I am now about to do. I can't wait for the day when I will truly understand why I have been so blessed. I will be forever grateful.

"Valen Cover

"Proud kidney transplant recipient of 8/13/02."

14

The Time of Her Life

"I have given up trying to understand life.
I am just going to live it."
—*Valen Cover*

Valen was well on the road to recovery following her August 2002 transplant, but as Tom Cochrane sings, "Life is a Highway," and for Valen there would be plenty of twists, turns, and dangerous curves to maneuver as she steered toward a new path in her life. There were no actual roadblocks—the word does not exist in her vocabulary. Some of the obstacles ahead were minor bumps along the way, while others were major potholes.

One annoyance occurred when she was visiting a friend in West York and parked her car in an alley. Inside the vehicle, on the floor, was her medicine bag containing a three-month supply of her vital medications and a backpack containing some clothes and CDs. When she returned to the car a short time later, the car had been broken into. Gone was the medicine bag, the clothes, and the CDs. It was important that Valen take her prescription drugs five times a day at precise times in the morning, afternoon, and evening. Luckily, the theft occurred after 10:00 p.m., giving a panic-stricken Valen and her mom time to renew the prescriptions overnight in time for the 8:00 a.m. medication. Pam remembered it as a difficult and scary time as she drove to a Baltimore drugstore in the middle of the night to replace her daughter's medicine. Police later recovered the clothes in a back alley, but they never found the drugs or the thief.

One of the first barriers to progress occurred when Valen was working full-time in November 2002 at the company where her father works. She was highly susceptible to germs, because she was immune-deficient and was taking an extremely high dosage of immunosuppressant drugs. She contracted the flu several times in her first month of work. She gave up the idea of permanent work until June 2003, and she has been working full-time ever since. Today, the good days outweigh the bad in terms of her health. She has had issues with medications she was taking, and in November 2003, doctors found pre-cancerous cells on her cervix. Her decreased immune system's response leaves the door open for them.

In August 2003, while working at Gerhardt USA, she met a man she liked. The six-foot-four gentleman asked her out, they began dating steadily, and he proposed to her on November 26th of that year. They were married on August 28, 2004. But it was not a marriage made in heaven. The union would last just over two years.

Valen has also attempted to make amends with her thirty-one-year-old brother, Brandon. They were close, growing up. When she separated from her husband in the summer of 2006, Brandon lived with her, and she enjoyed hanging out with her brother.

But they became distant for several months at the end of the year, and the sibling relationship became strained. I had a respectful and enlightening half-hour chat with him while doing research for this book. He said his life is complete and he is happy. He also shared with me the pain he felt for his sister's medical troubles. "I would not wish that on anyone. I have passed PKD on to my son, Branson, and when I looked at Valen during her illness it was like looking into a mirror of my future."

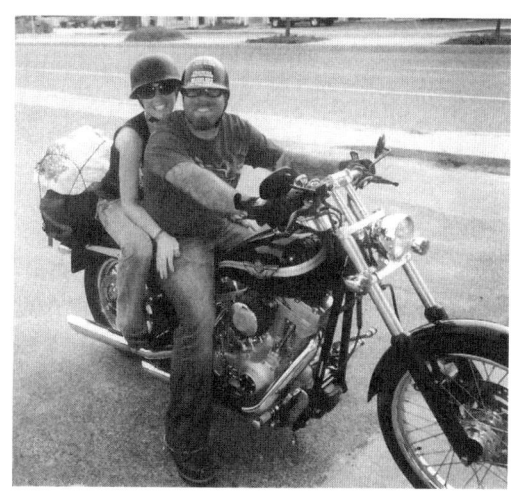

Brandon and Valen heading home from a beach trip to Ocean City, MD, in 2006.

Brandon said he suffers daily pain, occasional kidney cyst bleeds, and infections. "My days are numbered," he said, without a trace of self-pity. "I have about ten years before my PKD problems become bigger than they are today."

He works by day for General Dynamics Corporation. And he has found love. He met Emily through Valen. Yes, Emily—Valen's former college room-mate and Sally's oldest daughter! The pair was married on April 12, 2008. Valen was a bridesmaid.

Shortly after I spoke with Brandon, Valen invited him to dinner, and Pam visited her son at his new home. All agreed that his marriage to the daughter of the woman who gave her kidney to Valen "completes the circle."

Valen's involvement with the PKD Foundation began in March 2004. She had known that it is the only organization in the world dedicated to finding a treatment and a cure for the devastating disease and she wanted to become actively involved in its good work. "I had an overwhelming desire to do some good in my life" she rationalized. "I checked out the Web site for the PKD Foundation, saw there is a chapter in Maryland, and I contacted the chapter coordinator."

The seed was planted. For the next four years, she would dream of one day devoting all of her efforts and energy to working for an organization that offers hope for a cure to kidney disease.

Valen jumped into her volunteer activities with both feet and hit the ground running. She was informed there had never been a PKD chapter in York or central Pennsylvania and would she consider forming a chapter. They had asked the right woman!

Her first project was to plan a fundraising walk for September 18, 2004, to coincide with the foundation's annual national walkathon to raise funds and awareness of the disease. Valen dove into her task, calling people and making arrangements for food donations, entertainment, prizes, custom T-shirts, park location, and permits. All of her efforts were performed after work, usually late at night, and on weekends.

A large part of the job involved generating publicity for the chapter, in general, and for the upcoming walk, in particular. She contacted the local media and arranged for interviews. On July 5, 2004, a feature story appeared in *The York Dispatch* under the heading "A spark of hope offered: Transplant patient starts support group." Valen was pictured holding a poster showing a kidney with polycystic disease and a healthy kidney. The article by *The York Dispatch* reporter, Megan Shirey, nicknamed the spirited PKD spokesperson: "Valen 'Sparkplug' Cover."

"Sparky" went on a media blitz, securing valuable — and free — newspaper space on behalf of her South Central Pennsylvania PKD Chapter, in various local media. Among the ink she got was a feature story and photo in the *York Sunday News* by "Health

Pulse" columnist Heather Pulse, on August 29th. That same month, 36,785 copies of *York Community Courier* carried an article about Valen's efforts to educate people about the disease and promote her Walk for PKD.

She didn't limit her promotional efforts to the media. One evening prior to the walk, Valen spoke to thirty-three members of the Stewartstown Lions Club, most of whom had never heard of PKD and certainly were not aware that it affects more people than Down's syndrome, cystic fibrosis, muscular dystrophy, and sickle cell anemia, combined. Following Valen's presentation, they knew all about it—as well as Valen's experience with the disease.

As the September 18th walkathon date approached, Valen was getting excited about her first organized Walk for PKD. She had collected an e-mail contact list of some 300 names; the organizational meetings were completed; the volunteers were in place; and Valen and her participants and sponsors were ready to hit the Heritage Rail Trail in York's County Park for the five-kilometer walk.

Then the storm arrived!

Sheets of rain became a torrential downpour. It was Hurricane Ivan! The rain caused flooding and the floods created mudslides. York firefighters closed the road to the park and forced the PKD participants to evacuate the area. Valen looked at the horse trailer filled with prizes and the donated items. She was disheartened. "I stood in the parking lot in the pouring rain and I was told I'd have to leave and cancel my event," she recalled three years later.

She was down but not beaten. Her spirits were not entirely dampened. The next day when she calculated the promised donations and sponsorships, she realized that $23,200 was raised for the PKD cause—without even holding the event! Any lingering gloom she might have felt disappeared completely when she saw pictures of her and her organizers in a PKD newsletter, huddled in the teeming rain next to the horse trailer. Other photos on the page—some showing submerged cars—illustrated the havoc caused by the storm. One photo caption read: "Even a hurricane couldn't keep these Walk for PKD volunteers at home!" They say there is no such thing as bad publicity. Once again, Valen Cover had turned lemons into lemonade!

Undaunted, the chapter and walk coordinator set out to organize her second Walk for PKD and lost no time organizing committees and holding monthly meetings. When the next walk took place, on the third weekend in September 2005, the day was sunny and hot as fire—but no firefighters were required this time. Over 170 people showed up at John C. Rudy County Park to walk five kilometers and raise $31,750 for the national PKD Foundation.

By the time Valen organized her third walk, in 2006, she was becoming a veteran at the publicity-generating game. This time she recruited the support of none other than Senator Mike Waugh, Member, Senate of Pennsylvania 28th District, York County.

Senator Waugh was elected to serve as senator for the citizens of York County in November 1998. Prior to being elected to the state Senate, he served in the state House of Representatives for six years beginning in 1992. Through Valen's efforts, Senator Waugh introduced a resolution in the Senate to proclaim September 2006 PKD Awareness Month in Pennsylvania. That was not the end of his involvement. He invited Valen to appear on his television show titled *The Commonwealth Report,* which airs on White Rose Community Television (WRCT). The communications vehicle allows him an opportunity to share information and ideas with his constituents.

Valen and the senator filmed a Public Service Announcement to promote the September 16, 2006 Walk for PKD before settling in for a thirty-minute taped interview. Senator Waugh began the show by telling his viewers that he had met a young lady from York who suffers from a common ailment that can be fatal if not treated with a kidney transplant or dialysis. For the next half hour, a poised, polished, and professional Valen responded to questions from the senator and described her battle with the disease in a manner that was animated, educational, and entertaining.

The September 16th Walk for PKD was held under rainy skies. The event began with a senatorial kickoff as the Pennsylvania lawmaker welcomed the 200 assembled participants and got the show on the road after a local singer sang the national anthem. Valen's PKD chapter raised $38,500 that day.

Valen was fast becoming a star spokesperson for PKD and was emerging as its poster girl—literally. Her bright, smiling face and personal PKD story was now appearing on large, colorful posters; also in *Stories of Hope* pamphlets; in magazines; and other ads created by the PKD national office in Kansas City. In 2005/2006, Valen was

Over 170 participants take part in the second Walk for PKD that Valen organized at York's John C. Rudy Park.

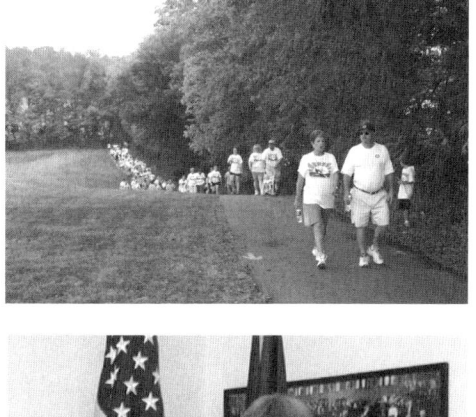

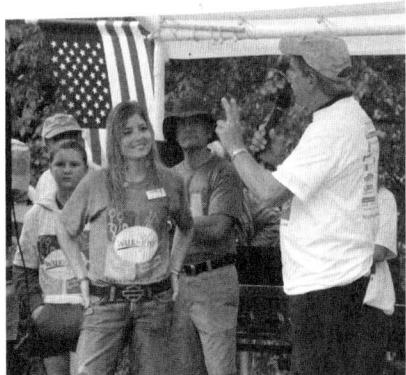

Senator Mike Waugh (white T-shirt) officially starts the third Walk for PKD that Valen organized.

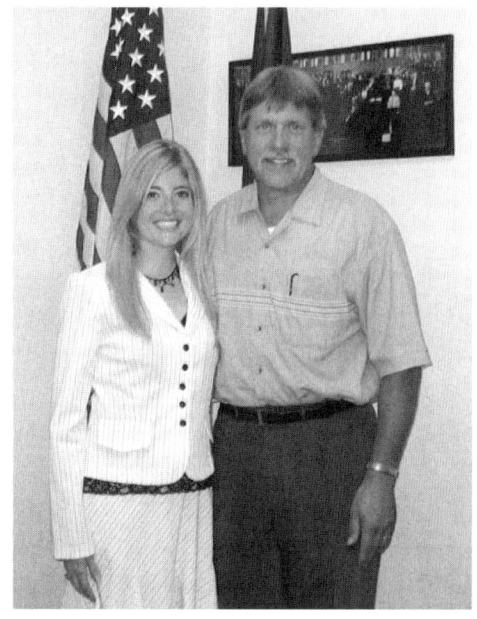

Valen first met Senator Mike Waugh in his office in 2006 when she recruited his support for a PKD Walk that she was organizing that year.

asked to chair the foundation's 12th Annual National Campaign for the Cure. The membership drive to 20,000 donors featured Valen's story as part of the effort to support PKD research, public awareness, and patient education. According to Dave Switzer, national director of marketing and public relations for the PKD Foundation, over $1 million was raised when Valen was Campaign Chair that year. Valen called it "a great honor" to serve as Chair of the annual campaign. The PKD Foundation, in its campaign material, countered that it was their "privilege to have such an encouraging and hopeful role model as Campaign Chair."

She was just twenty-two years old!

The young woman from York was also becoming a sought-after speaker and presenter at PKD conferences across the country. She attended the 16th Annual PKD Conference in Anaheim, California, in June 2005, and spoke to approximately 300 doctors, researchers,

PKD patients, and other delegates. She returned home to read in her hometown paper an article about her appearance as a guest speaker. A small, bold-face headline over the story and her photo noted that she had received a standing ovation following her presentation.

She spoke again at the 17th annual conference in Washington, DC, and also flew to Texas to be guest speaker and appear in a fashion show benefiting PKD. After addressing a luncheon gathering of some of the Lone Star State's finest ladies of fashion, Valen herself was invited to take part in the November 3, 2006, show at the Marriott Solana Hotel in Westlake, Texas, titled *Passion for Fashion*.

Her crowning achievement in public speaking may have come on March 30, 2007, when she summarized a poignant retelling of her life story at the Congressional Kidney Caucus on Capitol Hill, in Washington, DC. The briefing was sponsored by the PKD Foundation, and Valen was there with its president and CEO, Dan Larson. The briefing was attended by Congressional staffers from key House and Senate committees that deal with federal funding for disease research. A week later, she received a handwritten note from Dan Lara, government relations manager for PKD, that read: "Valen: A very big THANK YOU for your help with the Congressional Kidney Caucus briefing. Everyone raved about your emotional and inspiring story. I hope that we can call upon you in the future. Best Wishes, Dan Lara."

One of her favorite speaking assignments is a talk she has given several times to medical students at Johns Hopkins University School

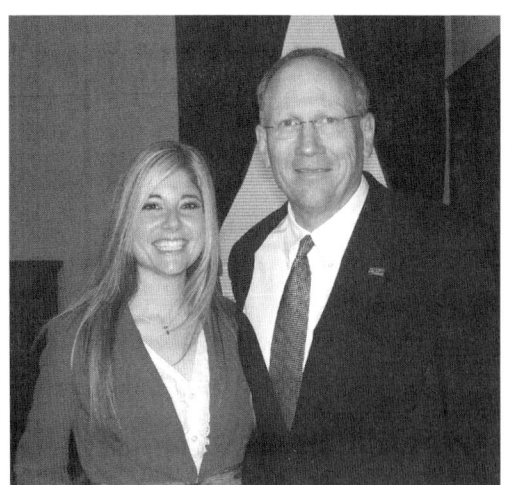

of Medicine. Each spring, for the past several years, she has talked about PKD to graduate students of Dr. Gregory Germino, Professor of Medicine at the university's Division of Nephrology and Professor in

Valen and Dan Larson, president & CEO of the PKD Foundation, speak on Capitol Hill, Washington, DC, at the March 30, 2007 Congressional Kidney Caucus.

the Department of Molecular Biology and Genetics. Dr. Germino, who is the husband of Valen's nephrologist, Dr. Terry Watnick, has called Valen "one of the greatest spokespersons for this disease who can relate to students who are around her own age." In a letter to Valen following her 2005 guest lecture, Dr. Germino wrote about her "tremendous enthusiasm, optimism, and hard work on behalf of the PKD community." He added: "The students really benefit by meeting someone so articulate and engaging." Valen is humbled by his comments. She is well aware of his stature in the medical community. One of his important contributions to the study of PKD include determining the genomic sequence of PKD1, its protein product, polycystin1, and the molecular mechanisms underlying the role of this gene in the development of the disease.

Valen's talk to the university students in 2008 took place during an auspicious week. She addressed the medical students just three days before her transplant surgeon, Dr. Robert Montgomery, led a team in the history-making six-way paired kidney exchange on April 5th at Johns Hopkins.

Among the many accolades Valen receives for her volunteer work on behalf of PKD, she treasures highly the handwritten notes from the people who work full-time for the Foundation educating the public, researchers, politicians, and medical practitioners about PKD and raising much-needed funds to help find a cure. From her portfolio of letters, she showed me one from Dan Larson thanking her for her "great session in Anaheim" and another from their PR and marketing executive, Dave Switzer, who sent a handwritten note to Valen thanking her for her efforts in making the 2005 Walk for PKD a success. He added: "Thanks for all you do — not only for the Walk — but for everything that is helping put PKD on the map."

Valen reached celebrity status within the PKD community when she was nominated for the first-ever DaVita.com National Kidney Idol Contest. The competition was sponsored by DaVita, Dialysis at Sea, and DaVita Patient Citizens. Dialysis at Sea is the largest provider of dialysis services aboard cruise ships in the world. Contest organizers wanted to hear uplifting, heartwarming and inspiring true stories about people in the chronic kidney disease or dialysis community who make a difference to those around them. Web site visitors were asked to nominate someone and write a 250-word story about their "Kidney Idol."

Thousands of people nominated kidney disease or dialysis patients, caregivers, friends, spouses, and health care professionals. An essay about Valen was chosen to be among four finalists. It was written by Lisa Dalto, a friend who is a volunteer with the PKD South Central Pennsylvania Chapter. Web site visitors then voted for the best of the four stories and determined that Lisa's story about Valen was the most inspirational. The prize was a seven-day cruise for two to the Eastern Caribbean aboard the luxurious Royal Caribbean International cruise liner. Valen enjoyed her first-ever cruise in February 2006.

When I asked Lisa Dalto why she nominated Valen, I soon realized it was a no-brainer.

"She is a wonderful friend and I admire and love her," was her initial response. Then she added: "Valen shines like she has a light within her soul."

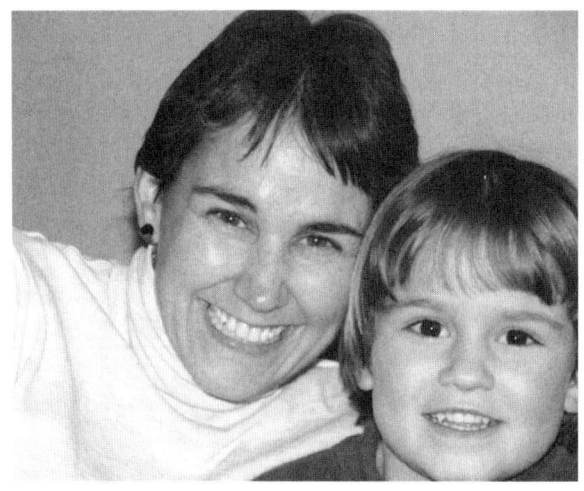

Valen's friend Lisa Dalto and her daughter, Paige, both have PKD.

Lisa lives in Hummelstown, Pennsylvania, with her husband, Dave, and their two daughters, Paige, six, and Claire, two. The family has not been immune to the devastation of PKD. Paige was tested at age two and has the disease. Lisa and Dave have not decided whether they will test Claire just yet. Lisa's paternal grandmother passed PKD on to her son, who passed it on to Lisa and her brother. Her brother has two children who have the disease. "Luckily, in our family, the disease seems to progress more slowly than with many other families," said Lisa, who turned forty-one in December 2007.

Lisa credits her parents for introducing her to Valen. They had become involved with the local PKD chapter and were encouraging Lisa to join. She was hesitant to commit to attending the meetings, but when her parents kept talking about the "amazing young woman" who ran the chapter, she sat in on a meeting because she was so intrigued by her folks' reaction to the chapter founder. "I met Valen at that meeting in the summer of 2004," Lisa related to me. "I was impressed by her humility, fervor, humor, passion, compassion, and leadership. She has that indescribable 'it' quality at such an early age." Lisa's 250-word essay in the DaVita contest summed up, perfectly, her feelings toward the "hard-working, genuine, seemingly tireless, young adult." She ended her nomination story by writing: "You will not leave her presence without knowing her gift."

Valen likes to say that life is hard but it's also wonderful.

A wondrous event for her occurred on the night of Friday, March 23, 2007, when a female acquaintance, Michelle, convinced her newly divorced friend to join her for a night at a popular York bar, The White Rose. Valen was not keen on doing the bar scene, but, to her delight, she saw a guy who caught her eye. They smiled at each other but did not speak. The next night both he and Valen showed up separately at another York bar. Valen believes it was a serendipitous occasion. "It was really weird, because both of us rarely go to bars, but on two consecutive nights we went to two different bars and saw each other both nights." That second night, they were watching and listening to the band, singly, but Valen could not keep her eyes off the good-looking, athletically built fellow she recognized from the previous night. "He has the best smile and eyes," she enthused. "I was hooked and I knew he was special."

Noah Keefer wondered why the pretty blonde was not drinking. Curious, the twenty-six-year-old asked her. "Because I have only one kidney," she told him, forthrightly.

"I felt like a jackass right out of the gate on that one," he told me several months later. "Strike one for me!"

Apparently, he got to first base that night because Michelle slipped Valen's phone number into Noah's hand as he was leaving the bar. Noah allowed an appropriate period of time to pass. Five days later, he called her on her cell phone. She was in Washington, DC, attending the PKD Congressional Caucus and preparing to deliver a briefing to the Congressional aides. Noah admitted he had never heard of PKD, so he got the *Reader's Digest* version on the phone "right then and there."

A recent college graduate and manager of a paint manufacturing company at the time, Noah admitted to Valen, a little facetiously, that he'd never met a woman who gave Congressional speeches in Washington. Her reply is now part of their folklore: "I'm not your average girl."

Valen smiles and attempts to vindicate herself whenever the now-classic line comes up in conversation. "This guy calls me and I barely know who he is, and when I said: 'I'm not your average girl,' I wasn't being snobby or setting myself on a pedestal, I just meant that I'm not average. I have, like, a million issues."

Needless to say, "this guy" was impressed. He asked her out. They met for dinner at Chili's, hit it off, and have been a serious item ever since. Several months after he met the "not-average" girl, I met the happy couple on a Saturday afternoon at the quaint, rented farmhouse they now share in Dover, outside York.

We sat at the kitchen table, and I asked Noah to tell me what he has learned about Valen since that initial phone call. "She is amazing!" he pronounced. "I soon found out what issues she was talking about, and now that I know, I am amazed how she dealt with them and became the positive person she is today."

Valen had left the room to search for a document upstairs that I had requested. Noah continued to speak freely of his feelings toward Valen: "I find it remarkable that there is absolutely no resentment towards anyone or anything. She is open and accepting of everybody. She really cares for people. She is truly remarkable."

As they got to know each other, they would uncover some enchanting coincidences that helped cement their relationship. A few weeks after they met, they were talking one evening in the living room of her apartment. When Valen mentioned going to her parents' home, Noah was a little startled when she mentioned the address. It wasn't that he was not keen to meet her folks; he revealed that he knew exactly where the house is located. "I worked at the garage right across the street from your mom and dad's home for two years, in 2000 and 2001," he revealed, astonishing both of them. "I used to park my car in the lot across the street right next to your car. Every day! And I'd see this sick young girl coming out of the house, from time to time." He now realizes that sick girl was Valen. He was too shy or embarrassed at the time to say hello, for fear of intruding on the family's anguish.

I instinctively knew I liked Noah the first time he offered me one of his favorite beers. Franziskaner's *weiss* products are top-fermented German beers that are noted for their zesty wheat flavor. But it took more than the refreshing taste sensation of an imported beer to convince me that he was the caring, understanding, sensitive, kind, and comforting individual that I'd hoped would come into Valen's life. For me, the first indication of his empathy towards Valen's "issues" came on August 13, 2007, when he announced to her that he was taking her to a special place on the fifth anniversary of her kidney transplant.

Valen doesn't like to save celebration for "special occasions." For the past four years, for example, she had celebrated her transplant anniversaries "only in my mind." She had told me more than once that every day was extraordinary for her. "Do not keep anything for a special occasion, because every day you live is a special occasion," she lectured me one time when I said I was waiting for a special occasion to call her.

Nevertheless, Noah convinced her to get dressed up in her finery for that evening. He took her to the Belvedere Inn Restaurant and Bar in Lancaster, Pennsylvania. Noah had been to the elegant inn previously, but Valen shared with me later that no man had ever taken her to such a nice place. She celebrated the occasion by enjoying the restaurant's signature king salmon, with spring vegetables and lobster risotto and mango buerre blanc. The next day, she covertly whispered to me on the phone that she didn't know how much the dinner cost. "But when he signed the check at the end of the meal, I noticed there was a 'one' in front of the total," she murmured.

For her part, Valen disclosed to me in early 2008 that she loves Noah and cannot imagine being without him. "My mother is my best friend and an extremely strong woman who taught me to never rely on anyone else for my happiness; that we can only find happiness within ourselves," she confided. "I agree with my mother's sentiment, but I also know that I have always longed for a strong, solid, secure, and healthy relationship, and that's what I have in Noah. He has made me a better person because he completes me and has helped to create incredible happiness in my life." Eight months after meeting him, she said she has been waiting her entire life for him. "We are so alike in so many ways, and we complement each other," she continued. "He is the guy version of me and I am the girl version of him." She chuckled at this last remark but turned serious again. "I believe it is important for two people like us to care for each other, equally. And I believe that we care about and love each other equally."

At this stage of her existence, now in her mid-twenties, Valen is convinced that she is in the strongest and most mature relationship of her life. "I feel like I am where I belong when I am with him and I look forward to whatever the future has in store for both of us."

Valen and Noah do many things together. They traveled for a week to California and they hike and even enjoy the simple activity of shopping together for groceries and household items. But her new adventuresome spirit allows her to fly solo once in awhile. And when given the opportunity, Valen does not glide, she soars. She found inspiration in a poem that is displayed at the Emig Mansion, where she and Noah stayed one night. It is titled *Faith Poem*, by Patrick Overton: "When we walk to the edge of all the light we have, and take that step into the darkness of the unknown, we must believe that one of two things will happen; there will be something solid for us to stand on, or we will learn to fly."

She took a small leap of faith in October 2007, when she signed up for the twelve-week Dale Carnegie Course. By the time the last Tuesday evening class wrapped up on January 22, 2008, Valen had received four public-speaking awards.

The Dale Carnegie Course teaches a wide range of effective communication and human relations skills, from public speaking to winning friends and influencing people. Valen proved to be a shining star among the group of forty-one in the class. On nights when every student is required to deliver a short speech, everyone receives a ballot and votes for the best speaker at the end of the evening. On November 6, 2007, Valen spoke about watching her transplant doctor perform a transplant operation on October 2nd. When the last of the forty-one two-minute speeches concluded, a vote was taken, and Valen received the "Outstanding Performance Award" by her peers. The next month, on December 4th, her speech to the class dealt with her successful efforts to "patch things up" with her brother, Brandon, who had been temporarily estranged from the family. She talked about initiating a meeting with Brandon in an effort to "break the ice and renew communication with him and our family." Her brief oration was judged the best of the night and she won the "Human Relations Award."

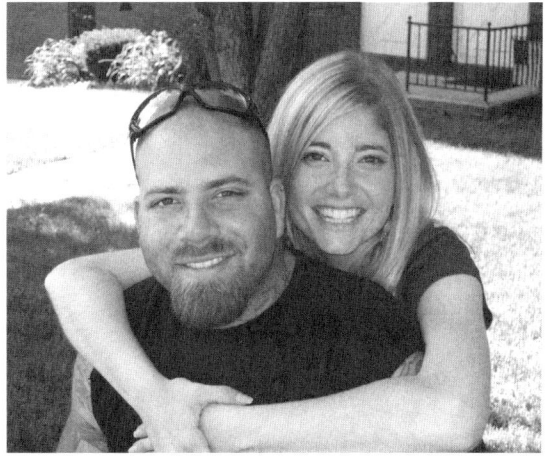

Valen gives her brother a hug outside the rented apartment they shared in the summer of 2006.

She wasn't finished collecting the gold! At the January 15, 2008, next-to-last class, she was named Human Relations Champion in a two-minute presentation that required each student to relate a specific incident that occurred since the start of the program and which applied Dale Carnegie's Human Relations Principles. The challenge was to provide a personal illustration that represented an effort to win friends and influence people. Valen chose to talk of a situation that had occurred that very morning. She was at Johns Hopkins Hospital to undergo a biopsy for pre-cancerous cells on her cervix. She has been doing this since 2003 and admitted she rarely speaks to anyone before, during or after the procedure, preferring to get the job done and get out of there in the shortest time possible. This time, however, she smiled at the doctor and nurse and struck up a conversation with them. "This led me to talk about my biography being written," she told me the next day. "The nurse was fascinated with my story and before I knew it the visit was over before I even realized it. Just as I was leaving, the nurse gave me a huge hug, squeezed my arm and said to 'keep looking up,' because God has a plan for me."

On the last night of classes, the Highest Award of Achievement is presented to the participant who, in the opinion of the other classmates, best exemplifies the standards, qualities, and principles on which the program is based. It is the most prestigious award of the program and is a tradition that began in 1912 and continues to this day. Students were encouraged to invite family members to the last class and listen to the short speeches. Bill and Pam were there to hear their daughter speak of the near-abortion incident and how just one person—in this instance, the little girl who locked eyes with Pam—can make a difference. It was a story with a happy ending, because, Valen told her classmates, her loving parents—who are her best friends and role models—have been by her side her entire life "just as they are tonight." After receiving the prestigious award on this final night, Valen told her father that she was humbled, honored, and in awe that her fellow students and peers would recognize her as best in the class, overall.

The next day she received an affectionate e-mail from her proud father. Valen shared it with me, with permission from her dad. This is part of what he wrote:

> Good Morning Valen,
> Once again you have given me and your mother more wonderful memories. Words cannot begin to express how very proud we are of you! I am inspired by the positive influence you have with people and how they truly believe you are someone who will have a positive impact on the lives of those you touch. I also believe this. It is very rewarding for me to watch you grow into the beautiful and special person you are, and to think that I played a minor role in who and what you have become. You are definitely on a roll! Stay in tune with yourself, continue to respect your health and the gift of life you were given, and go for the gold!
> With teary eyes and love,
> Your Father.

Valen responded with a grateful message to her dad. "A night like last night is living proof that the pain we endured has given strength to others," she wrote. "It is comforting to know that our family has turned our pain into positive energy and we are helping to make a difference in people's lives. For me, it sheds light on the suffering we have endured and it provides closure on some of the pain of the past." Her letter of love went on to give credit to her mother and father who are "fully responsible for me becoming the woman I am. It is because of you and Mom that I was able to overcome extreme health issues and now I thrive on inspiring others. If it were not for you, Mom, and Sally, all of this would not be happening."

15

The Letter From Noah

"From the young to the elderly to the young-at-heart,
she is an inspiration to all."
— *Noah Keefer, in a letter about Valen.*

Valen met the man she calls "the love of her life" on March 23, 2007, and the two have been inseparable ever since.

Nearly a year after their happy-chance meeting in a York bar, I asked Noah Keefer if he would consider outlining his feelings about Valen in a letter to me that I could include in this book. The dashing Romeo agreed and stoked the flame of his passion by writing the letter below about his Juliet:

> Meeting Valen has changed my life forever!
> I realize I am not alone in saying this, because when I hear people talk about her, from the young to the elderly to the young-at-heart, she is an inspiration to all.
> I have known Valen for just a year, but it feels like I have known her all my life. She is the type of person that makes people want to become the best they can. When she looks at you with that big smile and those beautiful, kind eyes, it is to know something spectacular.
> I have never met anyone like her before, and I know I never will again because this type of luck comes only once. She has forever changed my perspective on love and life. I love the way she is always scanning things; taking in the simple pleasures of life that most of us miss and have forgotten to see. It makes me step back and realize how truly wonderful life is.
> I am a picky person, so I have been told, in both life and love. I am quick to find something in most people that I don't like about them, something that would keep me from having them as a best friend, or pursue a serious relationship with. I have not found anything like this in Valen. From every freckle

on her face, every scar on her body, her every thought, there is nothing that can make me think she is anything but perfect. Perfect for everyone? No! But for me, she has awed me the way no one has ever come close to doing.

She is the person I could see spending the rest of my life with. I would constantly try to repay the way she makes me feel: as she falls asleep in my arms, as she smiles at me, as I appreciate her little idiosyncrasies that I had forgotten to appreciate in this truly wonderful life.

It is strange how we can know people our entire lives that have no impact on who we are and who we want to be. Then, we meet someone who changes our life and how we will lead it forever. Valen has been that person for me: a life-changing inspiration and a person that I love with all my heart.

I can't wait to see what the future has in store for us so I can try to repay this gift she has bestowed upon me.

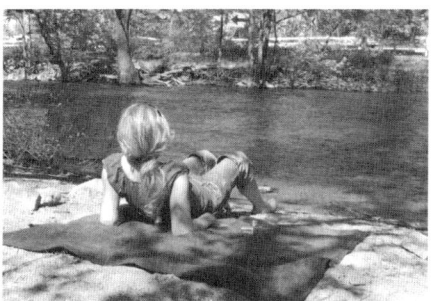
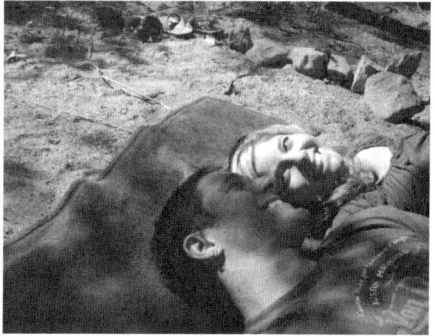

Valen loves the water, so Noah snapped this picture of her in a contemplative mood by Yellow Breeches River, a favorite spot of theirs near Dillsburg, PA.

Self-portrait taken at Yellow Breeches.

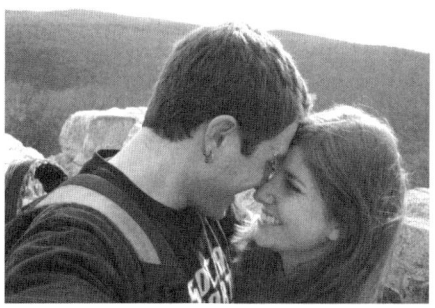
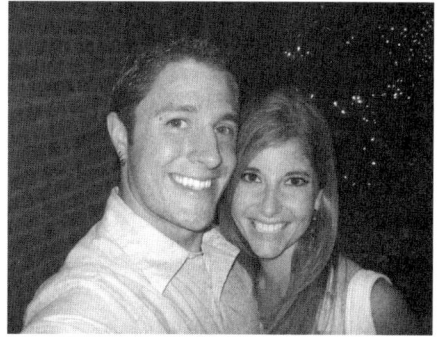

A "nose kiss" after hiking to the top of Chimney Rock, part of Catoctin Mountain in the Blue Ridge Mountains.

Valen and Noah celebrated at the Belvedere Inn Restaurant, in Lancaster PA, on the night of Valen's fifth anniversary of her kidney transplant.

16

The Questions
and the Answers

"All my life I've been harassed by questions."
— *Luis Bunuel, Spanish filmmaker*

Throughout my career it has been my job to ask questions. Since the early 1970s, I have interviewed a countless number of people for hundreds of articles that have appeared in over sixty-five publications around the world.

Valen ranks among some of my best interview subjects: intelligent, confident, articulate, and witty. Very witty! One Saturday night, a group of us were eating on the patio of T.J. Rockwell's American Grill & Tavern in Elizabethtown, Pennsylvania. I had put Valen Elizabeth Cover through the question grinder that day, interrogating her with queries about her life, ranging from the mundane to the momentous. Before our meals arrived, we were all enjoying some drinks. Her dad and I were sampling a Sea Dog Blueberry Wheat beer, and Noah was quaffing an ABC Water Gap Wheat. No one was slaking his or her thirst on a Rolling Rock beer, that great pale lager founded in Western Pennsylvania, but Valen had us rocking and rolling with laughter as she raised her bottle of Corona beer into the air and performed a rollicking good impersonation of me. Reverently holding the bottle in the air—as a priest would elevate a communion host—she turned and twisted it in her hands, studied it from various angles, and asked herself a philosophical question, dubbing it a "Dennis Question." She lowered her tone of voice: "Okay, Valen, in the grand scheme of your life, what exactly does this bottle of beer mean to you?"

I wouldn't recommend that she take this act on the road, but it was good. Achingly good. I had been on the delightful receiving end of what she likes to call her "smart-ass humor" many times, but this comedy routine/imitation was a side of her I had not witnessed previously. It also made me realize that the more I get to know Valen E. Cover, the more I know there is a lot I do not know about her, if you know what I mean.

So, in an effort to shed more light on the subject, I put myself "in the know" by posing more than twenty questions to this enlightening young woman, some months later. Here are my queries and the replies that she offered in early 2008:

DENNIS: *What makes you happy?*

VALEN: I absolutely adore children, and I love meeting new people and providing inspiration to those who need it most. I thrive on challenges and I enjoy conquering new things. I love spending time with my parents and I absolutely adore seeing them happy. I have seen too many days of sadness on their faces; fear in their eyes; and broken hearts. Today, seeing their warm eyes and happy smiles brings more joy to me than words can justify. My parents are now happier than they have ever been and enjoying life like never before. For me, that is the best feeling, because even though I was a good child, my health issues turned their lives upside down for so many years. It brings tears to my eyes to talk about them because that is how much I love them. All I want to do is make them proud.

D: *What makes you sad?*

V: Imagining a life without my parents. The thought scares me. I hate the prospect of my mom becoming ill with PKD.

D: *Who inspires you?*

V: My parents. I am sorry that all of my answers seem to revolve around them but they are my rock. They mean the world to me. They are determined, motivated, and successful people and those qualities inspire me. I tend to get inspiration from all of the positive-thinking people in my life that I love and adore. I actually try to find inspiration in everyone I

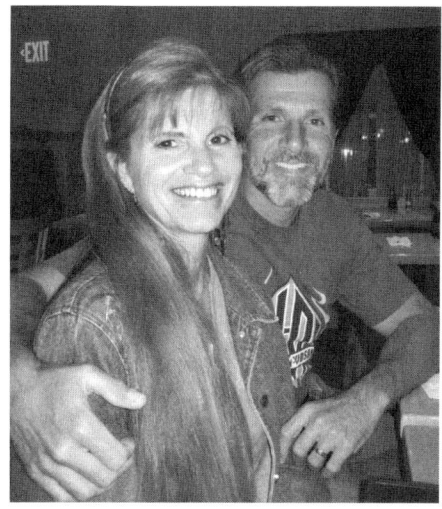

Valen's biographer took this picture of Pam and Bill at a dinner in August 2007 at Masa, a York sushi restaurant.

meet and take away something positive from every single encounter because I truly believe that we all can be inspired by every single person we meet.

D: *What do you look for in a friend?*

V: I like friends who are honest, not envious of others, and fun, because I love to have fun!

D: *I probably know the answer to this, but who's your best friend?*

V: My very best friend in the world is my mom! She is genuine and giving, and everything she does is in my best interest. I rarely ask her for anything, but she will drop everything to do anything for me, without hesitation. My dad is also my best friend. I can tell him and Mom anything. They have devoted so much of their time and energy to raising and taking care of me and now I just want them to enjoy each other and enjoy life! Dad has always been there for me and has always wanted to be part of everything that goes on in my life. Just before Christmas 2007, he and I took the train to New York City for the day to experience the Christmas festivities in that amazing and vibrant city, for the first time. We ate at an Irish pub; walked to Central Park, and along Fifth Avenue; saw the big Christmas tree at Rockefeller Center; went to Times Square; and stopped at a Starbucks. We had a nice dinner at AJ Maxwell's Steakhouse at 57 W 48th Street, and came home. Just me and my dad. It was a fun time.

D: *What do you want most in life?*

V: To be healthy and happy. I sometimes think that I would like to be remembered for all time, but I would be happy living a

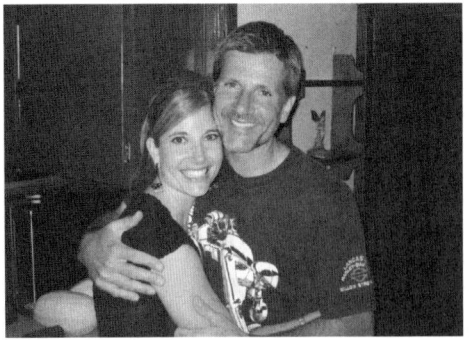

Bill gets a hug on his fifty-first birthday at the farmhouse that Valen and Noah share.

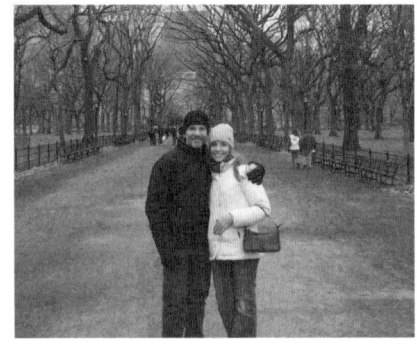

Valen and her father in New York's Central Park, December 2007.

simple life, working in a meaningful job; maybe live in a little house by the water with a wonderful companion, and children who are PKD-free.

D: *You are never without your pink cell phone. How important is it to you?*

V: Besides making and taking calls, I use it for text messaging, checking my schedule on the datebook, and taking pictures with it. I don't have a landline at home, so it's my best means of contact with the outside world. I'm not so petty as to say it's my lifeblood, but it is important to me. I have actually left the house without it a few times. It didn't even faze me. But you never know when I'm going to get that life-altering phone call. ☺

D: *You once said your hair is important to you. Tell me about it.*

V: I like to wear my hair long, but I wish I could have the hair I had in high school when it was thicker, longer, richer, and healthier. But that will never happen again, because of the damage done to it by dialysis, the medications I am taking, and the motorcycle accident. The day after the accident, I ran my fingers through my hair and huge clumps of it came out. My head was so swollen; the hair follicles died and fell out.

D: *What is your favorite season?*

V: I like the fall with the changing colors of leaves on the trees. At that time of year, I like to wear jeans, flip-flops and a T-shirt and go out and enjoy the season. I don't like super-hot weather. Because of some of the medicine I take, like my blood pressure medicine, I feel dizzy in the heat and the meds could make me susceptible to skin cancer when I'm in the hot summer sun. I love the rain! I enjoy the peaceful sound of rain and I like to stand in it with my head to the sky. I find that cleansing. I love any body of water, from streams to rivers to the ocean. One of my favorite quotes (author unknown) is: "Life isn't about waiting for the storm to pass. It's about learning to dance in the rain."

D: *You like a good quote. What's another of your favorites?*

V: One that sums up my attitude is by that same writer, Author Unknown: "Our lives are not determined by what happens to us but by how we react to what happens; not by what life brings to us, but by the attitude we bring to life. A positive attitude causes a chain reaction of positive thoughts, events and outcomes. It is a catalyst, a spark that creates extraordinary results."

D: *What's your favorite holiday?*

V: I enjoy Christmas because I get to spend a lot of time with my family. When I was a child, Christmas was a magical time. I loved to wake up and run downstairs to see what Santa brought. As I got older, I enjoyed the fun our family had at that time of year. Family time is priceless and something I treasure. I never knew what to expect at Christmas, because I was usually sick. But despite that, I still enjoy the season. When I was deathly ill at Johns Hopkins, my parents decorated my hospital room for Christmas. They were trying to make my life as normal as possible, even if it meant decorating a hospital room! How painful that must have been for them! No matter the state of my health, we always made the best of Christmas, and Mom and Dad did everything to make it as wonderful as possible for me. It is ironic that my most memorable Christmases are the ones when I was ill and my parents found a way to celebrate. I believe at such low points in one's life, we can fully understand the real meaning of the season and the true value of family.

D: *What food do you like?*

V: How much time do you have? I love food and I eat healthily. My weight is between 110 and 115 lbs. It fluctuates because of the prednisone anti-rejection drug I am taking. After my transplant in 2002, I put on thirty-five pounds. I joined Weight Watchers, lost it all, and I have kept it off ever since. Having said that, these are some of my favorite foods: salad; fruit such as kiwi, pineapple, avocados, and strawberries; any cereal; most fish but especially Mahi Mahi, salmon, tuna wrap, and Tilapia; red meat only occasionally; Louisiana Hot Sauce; salsa; Mexican food; black bean burgers; sweet potato fries; peanut butter on banana or apple; carrot cake; ice cream; angel food cake with fruit; strawberry kiwi pie made by Noah's mother; and anything my mom makes, like chicken pot pie and Hog Maw, which is her recipe of potatoes, sausage and carrots stuffed and cooked in the lining of a pig's stomach. Oh, and I am addicted to sushi. Noah and I go to a restaurant in York called Masa, where I always order the Yellow Submarine, which is made of rice, smoked salmon, avocado, tomato, cream cheese, and a piece of mango on top.

D: *I like how you tease me with that well-known Canadianism, "eh?" but how come you spell it differently than everyone else?*
V: Ey?

D: *I also like some of your terms of endearment. You've called me a "goober" and a "dork," and once, when I expressed an irrational fear of something, you joked that I was a "chicken-butt." Name a few of your other favorite expressions.*
V: Fabulous. Knucklehead. Super-buzzin'. Babe. You're silly.

D: *What are your greatest fears?*
V: Being on dialysis again scares me. I am afraid that my health will hold me back from being a free spirit and prevent me from doing some of the things I want to accomplish in life, but I try not to dwell on that. It scares me that I might be one of those tragic figures you read about, like a young woman who has been through a lot, gave a lot back, and then died in some freaky way . . . like in a motorcycle accident!

D: *How is your health today?*
V: Overall I feel great! I work full time and I have lots of excess energy. My blood pressure is under control, but I have issues with my immunosuppressant drugs. Prednisone (a steroid) and Prograf lower my immune system so my body will not reject the kidney. But I have pre-cancerous cells on my cervix that won't go away. I hope they will never progress to cancer. I am very thankful for how good I feel on a daily basis and I keep my fingers crossed that my kidney will last a LONG time!"

D: *What medications do you currently take?*
V: Right after my transplant I was taking forty pills a day, but that number is down significantly. I take meds at 10:00 a.m., 2:00 p.m., and 10:00 p.m. every day. They include the anti-rejection drugs Prograf and Prednisone; Prilosec to protect the lining of my stomach due to the bleeding vessels and ulcers I had in the past. I take a cranberry supplement to help prevent urinary tract infections, which

could easily lead to a kidney infection; the supplement K-phos; a blood pressure medicine called Metoprolol; the supplement Magnesium; and Stress tab B-complex which is a common vitamin I have been taking since my transplant.

D: *How do you deal with pain and suffering?*
V: There are two different kinds of pain: mental and physical. I am fine, mentally, because I don't dwell on it. Physically, I just deal with the pain until it goes away. What choice do I have? When I was really sick, I would sometimes regard the pain as a challenge and when I got through it, I felt like I had conquered, or won, something. Basically, I just dealt with the matters at hand.

D: *What kind of music do you enjoy listening to?*
V: I like all kinds of music, depending on my mood. Jo Dee Messina's lyrics inspire me as does a beautiful song by The Wreckers called "Stand Still, Look Pretty." I listen to it when I'm sad. Even though the lyrics are depressing, it inspires me when they sing: *"You might think it's easy being me; you just stand still, look pretty."* I wonder if some people think that, when they look at me, but they have no idea of the scars underneath my clothes and the pain I have been through. Heavy metal is fun to listen to if I'm angry, but I don't like rap. Noah likes the punk band Social Distortion, and we saw them in concert in Allentown. That was fun. I like alternative music and I love country, but not the twangy kind, and also every type of girly slow song because I'm a girl. I took my dad to see Faith Hill and Tim McGraw in concert for Father's Day one year, and then he and I took Mom to see her favorite rock band, Aerosmith, in Hershey. They played her favorite songs, "Dream On" and "Fly Away From Here."

D: *What are some of the more memorable movies you have seen?*
V: I like movies with a good story, like *Good Will Hunting* with Robin Williams and Matt Damon, and I have seen *Stranger Than Fiction*, with Will Ferrell, twice. It's about a guy whose life changes dramatically when he starts to hear his life being chronicled by an author only he can hear. I love the way the story is a mix of fiction and reality and that it shows how one tiny decision or event in your life can change everything. Every seemingly insignificant thing we do leads us to where we are today and where we are going

tomorrow. Every decision in life matters. The character, IRS Agent Harold Crick, changes his life and finds love when he discovers that the book being written about him might kill him. The movie makes me think of my life.

I tend to be attracted to movies about sick people, like *A Walk to Remember*, which is about an eighteen-year-old girl, Jamie, in a small North Carolina town, who is dying of leukemia. At one point, she tells her distraught boyfriend, Landon: "Without suffering there would be no compassion." And as Jamie lay dying, she says: "Maybe God has a bigger plan for me than I had for myself." There is a quote in that movie that I love. Jamie knows she is dying and she does not want to fall in love with Landon. She said she does not need a reason to be angry with God.

Another movie I like is *Here on Earth*, a romantic story of friendship and true love. The dialogue is very touching, especially when the girl's father says to her: "It's good to be your father," and she replies: "It's good to be your daughter." Simple, but heartwarming. I also love the poetry of Robert Frost, and there are some great lines in the movie from Frost's poem, "Birches": *"I'd like to get away from earth awhile; And then come back to it and begin over."* Another movie I loved is the 2008 film *Juno*, starring Canadian actress Ellen Page. In one scene, sixteen-year-old Juno is asked what she is doing and she replies that she is dealing with things way beyond her maturity level. That's the story of my life!

D: *In* A Walk to Remember, *Jamie has a list of all the things she wants to do in her life. What are the top three things on your list?*

V: 1.) I would like to get married again and have a relationship and family as solid as the one I have with my parents. I would like to have a child, even though it could be detrimental to my health and a challenge in my life. I sometimes think it would be best for me to not have a child, but then I think I would like to provide a child with the kind of love and relationship I share with my parents.

2.) I want, somehow, to repay my parents for everything they have done for me. I don't know how possible this is, but I want to.

3.) After I am gone, I would like to be remembered for the lives I have touched. I want my story to live on so I can still be doing good things and changing lives for the better, even when I'm no longer here.

17

The Testimonials

"Valen is a woman of strength who is leading others with her determination and courage. She is blessed to be a person who inspires, encourages, and gives hope."
— Lisa Dalto, Volunteer, PKD Chapter,
South Central Pennsylvania

When Valen graciously agreed to allow me to write her life story, I warned her that I would not portray her as the next Mother Teresa. She agreed, adding that if I represented her as St. Valen there'd be hell to pay. I hope I have not done that. I don't have any "burning" ambitions!

I also made it clear to her that I have no intention of ever writing her obituary, as I did for our friend Ed Loch. I expect to be biding my time in God's Waiting Room at some Retired Writer's Residence on a South Sea island long before she makes her worldly exit. Every picture has a story and every story has a beginning. Every story should also have an ending. Except this one. I truly believe Valen's story is a never-ending one. I kidded her that I will update her biography every twenty-five years. Give or take.

Since you've read this far, you know what I think of Valen Elizabeth Cover. I wanted to find out what others—outside of her family and the medical community—think of her, so I asked ten people who know Valen well. I asked a childhood friend, a boss, a colleague, a state senator, high-school friends, and others to tell me their "Valen Story."

It's a good thing I limited the number to ten. I received thousands of words of praise. Mark McGuire, an admirer of Valen's since childhood, wrote six pages of commendations and reminiscences in three separate e-mails. Bob Galloway, her former boss at Lincoln General and a family friend, wrote a letter containing 2,001 words (Thanks, *MS Word* count!). I joked with him that he should have added one more word to make it a significant number (Valen had her transplant in 2002).

Here are the edited versions of the bouquets they offered (including Lisa's at the start of the chapter):

Senator Mike Waugh
Member, Senate of Pennsylvania
28th District, York County

"Valen impressed me with her sincerity and dedication. She doesn't complain or feel sorry for herself. Valen is working to bring about a cure that will not only help her but others who suffer from this condition (PKD)."

Bob Galloway
Family friend and Valen's former boss at Lincoln General

"It is redundant to say that Valen is wonderful and unique but we know it to be the truth. I have known Valen and her family for over three years and have had the pleasure to be with them on several long motorcycle rides, both socially and for charitable causes. It's a real treat at the end of a ride to enjoy a good meal but especially to see Valen abandon her strict diet and enjoy the momentary pleasure of a large serving of sweet potato fries. The motorcycle accident in May 2007 set her back, but not much. Through determination and commitment, she threw herself back into a life that focused on her family, PKD volunteering, work, and friends.

"In her job, I like that she works diligently, completes projects effortlessly and enthusiastically, exhibits a professional appearance and proper work ethic, and helps create a pleasant atmosphere for the rest of the staff. She is extremely accomplished in administrative skills and project coordination, but I don't want this to sound like a job resumé. I would rather talk about the influence she has on young people, especially at the PKD Walks she has organized. I took part in the September 2007 walk and while on the bus that took participants to the start of the route, I overheard some of the passengers talking. One little girl asked her mother: 'Will I get to see Valen?' Later, during the walk through the fairgrounds, I heard more children exclaiming to their parents: 'I got to talk to Valen!' and, 'Isn't Valen nice?' As I observed the faces of the children and their parents—many of whom were PKD victims—I could see that Valen was offering hope and encouragement through her personal struggle and ultimate victory over the disease.

"I see three personas in Valen: One is a laughing teen-like girl who loves meeting people and visiting new places; precocious; concerned with her personal appearance; a little naïve, perhaps; but always seeking new adventures. Another persona is a very confident young woman; extremely intelligent; fun-loving, cares deeply for family and friends; dedicated to helping others—not just PKD sufferers, but anyone in need; and a person who is fully aware of her challenges and limitations because of her medical condition. The third individual I see is a very mature person; wise beyond her years; patient; one who perseveres; and is aware of a plan in life for personal and professional success. What sets her apart from so many others is her willingness to share herself with others for the greater understanding of life and for the benefit of all.

"Valen loves life and holds every moment as precious. All of us who know her are better people for knowing her and for having the opportunity to share our lives with her."

Von Trout
PKD victim, Carlisle, PA

"I have known Valen for over two years and I know you asked me not to call her 'wonderful and unique,' but those two words perfectly describe my feelings about her. She and I have more in common than our PKD, like our love of country music. When we met for the first time, we hugged like only a "cyst-er" could understand. She possesses a positive spirit and I try to live my life in the same way. That connects us."

Adam Shaub
High school friend, Pittsburgh, PA

"Mine was the first face Valen saw when she woke up from her transplant. I was rubbing her forehead to comfort her. I knew she was worried and scared; I just felt I needed to be there for her. I said something to make her smile. It was such a relief to see that beautiful smile. She has grown so much since I knew her in high school, despite her health issues. I have seen her frustrated and annoyed, but she never gave up. Ever! I think it's because she takes a proactive approach to everything. She never looks back. Ironically, she gives everyone else so much strength. She will change the world. She can do anything she puts her mind to. I believe in her 100%."

Dave Switzer
National Director, Marketing and Public Relations
PKD Foundation, Kansas City, MO
www.pkdcure.org
"Valen is an incredible woman who has done amazing things with her life and to help raise awareness of PKD. Despite the many health issues she has endured, her spirit and smile remain strong. She has a willingness to share her story with everyone, from reporters and members of Congress to people and families who must deal with this disease every day. Valen is a persuasive and inspirational voice in the battle against PKD."

Ashley Manfredo
High school friend, Pittsburgh, PA
"Valen and I were typical teenagers in high school, spending hours on the phone and choosing outfits for school the next day. If we weren't on the phone we were at each other's house. We were inseparable. She helped me find myself through those awkward teenage years. Even though we now live a few hundred miles apart, I can pick up the phone and talk to her like we never skipped a beat. I know I will always get her honest opinion, no matter my situation. We have seen each other through some rough times over the years. She has been my angel ever since the first time I met her. Her friendship is a priceless gift that I was granted and I will treasure it, always."

Sam Bashore
Friend, Harrisburg, PA
"Valen has an incredible ability to persevere through physical roadblocks in her life but I know she would much rather have spent a year in college than in the hospital! I see an incredibly strong young lady who refused to give up in her personal struggle. Her infectious smile covers a lot of her emotional scars. There was a time after her transplant when Valen was in the emergency room of the hospital with a high fever, which could be tantamount to a major illness for a person without a fully-functioning immune system. I

asked if she had called her parents and she said: 'No, they must not know!' She reminded me that her parents had been through enough with her PKD. For me it was a defining moment in her character: The child was making decisions for her parents! And that is where her inner strength comes from: her parents. Every quality you see in Valen exists within her parents.

"If you had never met Valen and talked to her without seeing her you would be hard pressed to determine if she was twenty-four or eighty-four. I say this because she has an above-average intellect mixed with a voice of directness developed from her traumatic experiences. She reminds one of a wise, older woman who can teach us many of life's hard lessons, but then you realize you are talking to a young, and in many ways, innocent lady.

"I believe the reason she has affected so many people in her community is due to the way she has decided to live the rest of her life. I have watched her consume every little experience of life with passion and excitement! It's as if she were blind her whole life, and now she can see!"

Randy King
Fellow transplant patient
Bethany Beach, DE

"Valen is a wonderful person and one of my heroes. I was a patient at Johns Hopkins the same time as Valen. We became friends in the hospital and remain good friends today. Dr. Montgomery performed Valen's transplant that wonderful morning of August 13, 2002, and he did mine that same afternoon."

Dick Mansberger
Service Department, Edwin L. Heim Company
Harrisburg, PA

"I met Valen through her dad, as he and I are both members of the International Brotherhood of Electrical Workers (IBEW) Local 29, York. I have watched her grow from a bright-eyed, innocent little girl to a mature, beautiful woman. Incredibly, she has not been jaded by her struggle with, and ultimate victory over, PKD. She has a sparkle in her beautiful eyes that readily invite you into her world. When she was very ill in the hospital, I visited her most Fridays and I witnessed Valen's magic many times. It is not an easy task to adequately express the essence that is Valen: She showed perseverance during what we have termed 'the hike from hell' to Lewis Rock in Michaux State Forest in humid, 96° F temperature. Unfortunately, she paid dearly for her persistence that day, for she suffered a seizure later that night. There is her tenacity, as revealed in her defeat of the devastating effects of PKD; there is her vulnerability, as seen when she requested a hug from every one of her hospital visitors; there is her compassion for fellow PKD sufferers as demonstrated by her volunteer efforts; there is her indomitable spirit that is evident in her upbeat take on life—no matter what dilemma she faces."

★ ★ ★

Valen used to ask herself two fundamental questions: "Why am I here?" and "What is my purpose in life?"

She thinks—at least, she hopes—she now knows the answer. "I overcame so much at such an early age, I wish with all my heart that my story will inspire and motivate others to appreciate life and never give up hope even when all seems lost. I never abandoned hope because we cannot survive without it. I want to help find a cure for PKD. This is the only sense I can make out of the years of devastation that my family and I have lived through, and I am determined to do whatever I can to make that happen! I have faith that I will live to see that miraculous day. My goal is also to help bring awareness to the importance of organ donation and the entire field of transplantation. I truly believe that one individual can make a difference. I encourage everyone to cherish life and live each day to its fullest and believe—with all your heart and soul—the words of Helen Keller: 'Life is an adventure or nothing at all.'"

Mandy Schwarz, Valen's former nurse at Johns Hopkins intensive care unit, spoke for everyone who knows and loves Valen Elizabeth Cover when she said, simply: "I look forward to her future."

18

The Cover Girl

"There were times she did not look like a human being."
— *Bill Cover*

Much has changed since Valen's deathly sick days, as referred to by her father in the above comment. As these photos confirm, so has her appearance, demeanor, and confidence. In 2007, two professional photographers shot a series of photos of Valen.

One session took place in a York photo studio and another at Loch Raven Reservoir in Baltimore. The photos here are a selection of several hundred images that were shot over two days. After taking over 400 digital pictures of Valen in various poses and settings, Baltimore photographer Maximilian Franz, whose work includes fine art photography, portraiture, and photojournalism, said simply: "You were born for this."

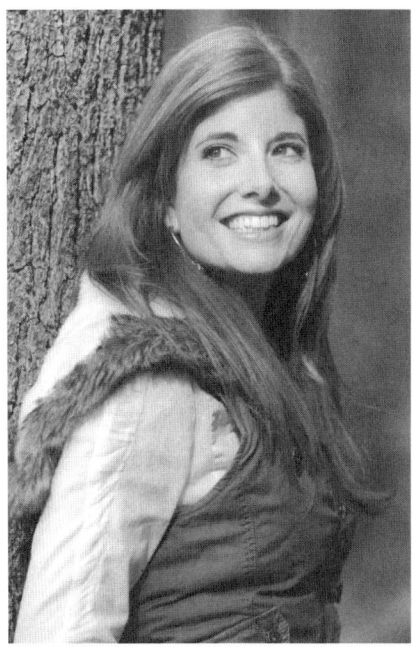 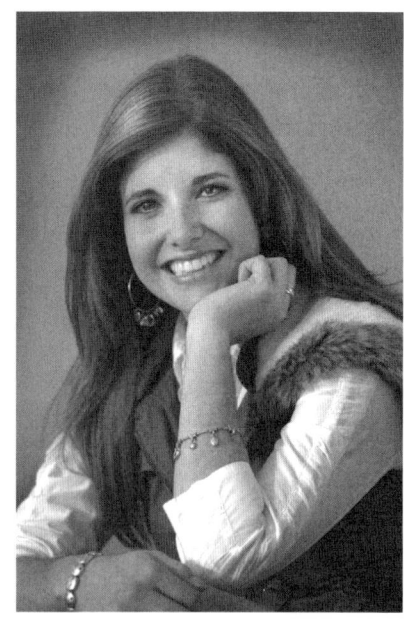

Photos by Maximilian Franz

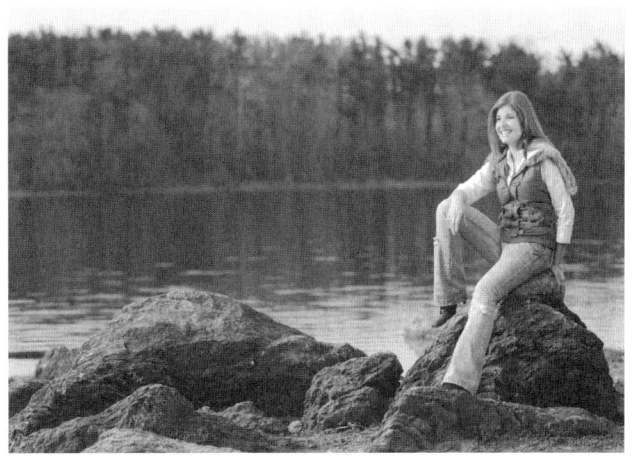

Photo by
Maximilian Franz

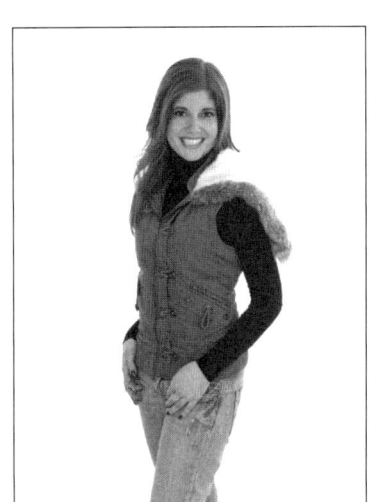

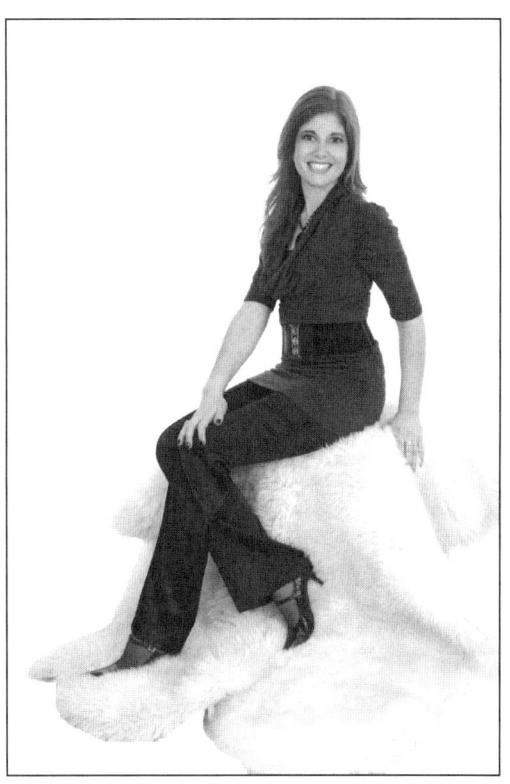

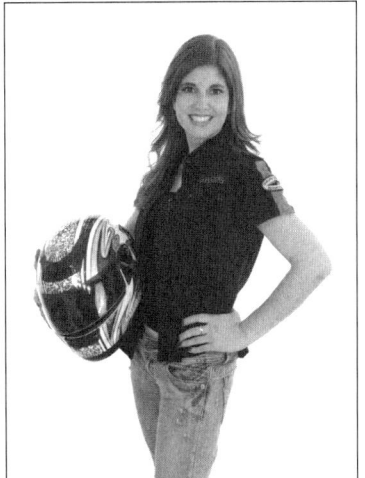

Photos by Byron Wilt

Acknowledgements

John Lennon once said that he put things down on sheets of paper and stuffed them in his pocket. "When I have enough, I have a book," he joked. That's basically what I did to produce this book. On one occasion, I didn't have a sheet of paper, so I used a Starbucks napkin.

It's a good thing I have "deep pockets," because I wrote down a lot of things about Valen Elizabeth Cover. It goes without saying that this book would not be possible if she had not shared her life story with me and granted me permission to share it with the world. She did so with the fervent desire that her story might offer inspiration, encouragement, and motivation to others who are lacking in faith and hope. I promised her that I would do my best to relay her message: "Despite all odds, things *can* get better. Never give up. Have faith. Miracles do happen!"

If Valen's mother had not been as openhearted, honest, and helpful as she was, I would have needed more than a miracle to write this book. Pam allowed me to delve into the darkest corners of her memory to learn the most intimate details of her daughter's battle against illness, disease, and accident. Pam has a keen inward eye, like a diary that she carries around in her mind. But she also shared with me the incredibly detailed *written* diaries, medical records, journals, and school documents that she has kept over the years. How else would I know that on the morning of Thursday, September 1, 1988, five-year-old Valen suffered a seizure, and for dinner that evening she had Lipton noodle soup while the rest of the family dined on leftover chicken corn soup?

Valen's father was also asked to walk down some dark hallways, open locked doors, and dredge up memories that he'd like to forget but cannot. It is said that sadness flies away on the wings of time, but on many occasions I swooped in on the Cover family and dug up details of their past, posing questions that I probably had no right to ask. I was overwhelmed by their cooperation, courtesy, and extreme kindness. I realize that what was hard to bear is certainly not sweet to remember. One evening, in the comfort of the home of Bill and Pam, I had the journalistic audacity to ask them to talk about some of the worst times of Valen's illnesses. Bill rose to the occasion and never once wavered. At times he responded to my probing questions with a powerful Churchillian eloquence; at other times he spoke very softly with the sensitivity of a father's love for a daughter he almost lost.

Valen, Pam and Bill are the three stars of this book, but it would not have seen the light of day without the help of many others too numerous to thank here. Most are mentioned in the book, such as the extraordinary and dedicated people who work at Johns Hopkins Hospital and in York medical centers. So many of them played leading roles in the telling of Valen's story, and, for me, it was humbling that they took so much time to talk to me about their beloved former patient. I devoted more than one chapter to Valen's kidney transplant surgeon, Dr. Robert Montgomery, because if he were a musician he'd be a huge rock star. His larger-than-life presence and contribution in the medical community cannot be overstated. His dedication and outstanding efforts in the field of kidney transplantation and in the development of a Paired Kidney Exchange Program **www.hopkinsmedicine.org/transplant/Programs/InKTP/ index.html** are among the most noble of human endeavors.

There is one other person who deserves top billing in the production of this book, and that is kidney donor Sally K. Robertson, who would prefer to shun the limelight; but without her precious gift to Valen, this book would not have been written.

There are many others, like Cinda ("Cindy") Grisbach, administrative assistant to Dr. Montgomery, who played important supporting roles, and to them I am grateful.

Thanks also go to the Cover family for opening up their photo albums and allowing me to rummage through pictures in search of childhood images of Valen and other members of her immediate and extended family. And to everyone else who supplied photos for the book: I thank you for your pictorial talents.

I am also grateful to Tim Gordon for publishing *My Favorite American*. Tim has published six other books of mine. That makes him My Favorite Publisher. His publicist Alison Roesler is one very delightful, down-to-earth, PR person; and editor Jane Karchmar is an extra-ordinary word polisher who also proved to be a wonderful and comforting cyber hand-holder, night and day. Her late night e-mails often soothed my tired mind as she wrote relaxing mantras, such as: "Don't worry, Dennis. It will get done and it will be good and it will come out just when it should." And to book designer Magdalene Carson: you make my words look good!

Last but certainly not least, I am indebted to my supportive wife of 32 years. Kris is my strength and the rock upon which I have built my career and my life.

About the Author

Dennis McCloskey has been a full-time freelance writer since 1980. A member of the Professional Writers' Association of Canada (PWAC), he earned a Journalism degree from Toronto's Ryerson University in 1971. He currently works as an independent corporate journalist and editor, magazine writer, and book author. Several hundred of his human interest and business articles have appeared in over sixty-five newspapers, consumer and trade magazines, and corporate newsletters in Canada, the U.S., and Europe. An avid traveler, he lives in the Greater Toronto Area of Richmond Hill, Ontario, Canada, with his wife, Kris, a schoolteacher. Visit Dennis at his Web site, **www.dennismccloskey.com**

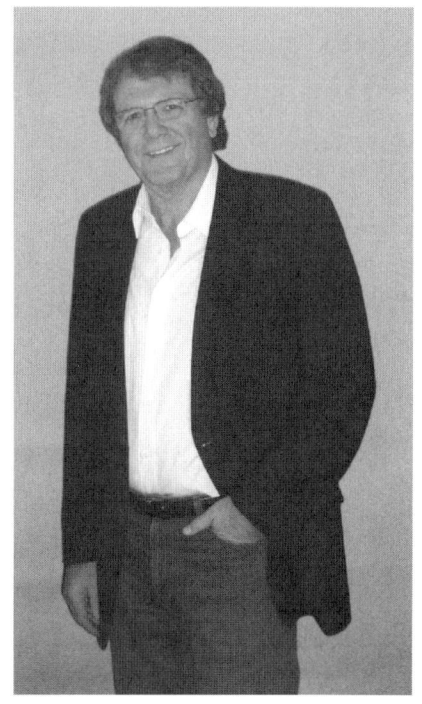

Photo by Jeff Davis

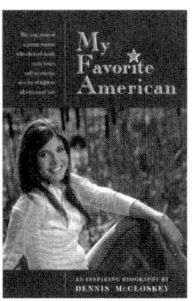
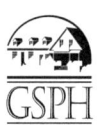